CARDIOLOGY RESEARCH AND CLINICAL DEVELOPMENTS

CARDIAC TAMPONADE

EPIDEMIOLOGY, CAUSES AND MANAGEMENT

CARDIOLOGY RESEARCH AND CLINICAL DEVELOPMENTS

Additional books in this series can be found on Nova's website under the Series tab.

Additional e-books in this series can be found on Nova's website under the e-book tab.

CARDIOLOGY RESEARCH AND CLINICAL DEVELOPMENTS

CARDIAC TAMPONADE

EPIDEMIOLOGY, CAUSES AND MANAGEMENT

CAMERON L. PITTMAN
EDITOR

NOVA BIOMEDICAL

New York

Library of Congress Cataloging-in-Publication Data

ISBN: 978-1-63482-787-4
Library of Congress Control Number: 2015938198

Published by Nova Science Publishers, Inc. † New York

Contents

Preface

Cardiac tamponade is a life threatening pericardial disease which is characterized by an obstruction of inflow of blood to the ventricles leading to a decrease of cardiac output as a result of the pressure around the heart caused by accumulation of fluid within the pericardial space in a sufficient quantity. In this book, the key elements of the anatomy and physiology of the pericardium are reviewed, and the pathophysiology, etiology, clinical features, diagnosis and management of cardiac tamponade are discussed. Regional blood flow and metabolic derangements reported in experimental models are reviewed as well. Other chapters examine the epidemiology, clinical presentation, diagnostic and therapeutic approaches of malignant pericardial effusion and a discussion of mood alteration (in particular, acute dysphoria) that is associated with cardiac tamponade, that which is widely mentioned in nursing and medical literature.

Chapter 1 – Cardiac tamponade is a life threatening pericardial disease which is characterized by increased pressure around the heart due to fluid accumulation in pericardial space which results in decrease in cardiac output. This condition is a medical emergency, and the complications of which include pulmonary edema, shock, and death. It is characterized by tachycardia, elevated jugular venous pressure, pulsus paradoxus, and hypotension etc. Electrocardiogram, Chest x ray and transthoracic echocardiogram are the key investigations that need to be done urgently to evaluate this clinical condition. Echocardiographically-guided percutaneous pericardiocentesis is the lifesaving procedure. Meanwhile, open surgical approach is also considered for traumatic cases, purulent pericarditis and recurrent malignant pericardial effusions. The overall mortality risk depends on the speed of diagnosis, treatment and the underlying cause of the tamponade. In this chapter, we will review the present knowledge of the etiology, pathophysiology, diagnosis and the management of cardiac tamponade.

Chapter 2 – The pericardium is composed of two layers – the visceral pericardium and fibrous parietal layer, and it contains a thin layer of fluid surrounding the heart. When larger amounts of fluid accumulate under pressure or when the pericardium is scarred and inelastic, one of three pericardial compressive syndromes may occur. Cardiac tamponade may be characterized by chronicity of fluid buildup and variant of pressure. Hemodynamic response in cardiac tamponade depends on the pressure in the pericardial sac and the ability of the heart to compensate for elevated pressure, which is directly related to the amount of fluid and the pericardial pressure-volume relation. With cardiac tamponade, all of the cardiac chambers are compressed due to increased pericardial pressure. Ultimately, cardiac chamber diastolic compliance is compromised.

Chapter 3 – Cardiac tamponade (CT) is a life-threatening clinical syndrome that requires timely diagnosis. CT is defined as a haemodynamically significant cardiac compression caused by pericardial fluid. The fluid may be blood, pus, effusion (transudate or exudate) or air and treatment involves correction of the cardiac diastolic restriction by removing pericardial fluid during either pericardiocentesis or thoracotomy. In CT systemic arterial hypoperfusion is followed by regional blood flow redistribution in order to preserve tissue and organ function. In this chapter we reviewed regional blood flow and metabolic derangements reported in experimental models. In the early stages of CT Portal venous flow reduction is associated with an increase in hepatic arterial blood flow, whereas in the late stage of low blood flow total hepatic blood flow is decreased despite redistribution between portal venous and hepatic arterial blood flow. The preservation of liver blood flow is due to a regulatory mechanism known as the hepatic artery buffer response (HABR).

In CT there are profound changes in the regional oxygen metabolism. Hepatic oxygen extraction reached values around 80%. Portal oxygen content became low due to an increase in mesenteric oxygen extraction during systemic low blood flow. Accordingly, in conditions of low portal blood flow, the HABR and redistribution of blood flow in the celiac trunk become critical for the maintenance of sufficient hepatic oxygen delivery. CT induces inadequate visceral perfusion which may interfere with integrity of the intestinal mucosal barrier and contribute to the development of multiple organ dysfunction. Gut luminal lactate increased relatively late during low systemic blood flow and could be explained by systemic hyperlactatemia. The proportional blood flow of the superior mesenteric artery was well maintained during progressive, severe CT and signs of systemic hypoperfusion preceded those of gut hypoperfusion. Signs of gut hypoperfusion (increased veno-arterial and mucosal arterial PCO_2 gradients as well as increased regional CO_2 content difference) preceded the signs of inadequate mucosal oxygen supply and the signs of gross jejunal wall dysoxia. Arterial blood lactate increased early during tamponade and was not explained by increased gut lactate release. Systemic hyperlactatemia is apparently due to lactate release from other tissues than the gut, but is also partly caused by decreasing hepatic clearance. Changes in lactate metabolism are not related to cell injury since Hepatic lactate extraction decreased, but hepatic release of glutathione Stransferase A did not change during CT. During low systemic perfusion, the HABR is exhausted and hepatic function is impaired without signs of cellular damage. Whole body venous efflux as an estimate of hepatic and extra-hepatic organ lactate efflux is of similar magnitude in hyperdynamic sepsis and in cardiogenic shock. In cardiac tamponade, regional, extra-splanchnic lactate production is accompanied by hepatic failure to increase oxygen extraction and net hepatic lactate output, despite maintained hepatic arterial perfusion. After CT it has been reported that vascular dysfunction persisted up to 6 h after release of tamponade. These inflammatory characteristics may also indicate that inflammatory activation is a possible pathway involved in the pathogenesis of cardiogenic shock. In a porcine model of acute splanchnic hypoperfusion, endothelin blockade restored hepato mesenteric perfusion and reversed lactate metabolism. These observations might be relevant when considering liver protection in low CO states.

Chapter 4 – Pericardium is a common site for neoplastic involvement that occurs due to direct local invasion by malignancy or metastatic spread via the lymphatics or bloodstream. Malignant involvement of the pericardium or occasionally treatment of malignancy can cause pericardial effusion. Pericardial effusion can be asymptomatic or cause chest discomfort, dyspnea, tachycardia, hypotension and cardiogenic shock, with increasing amount of fluid. Electrocardiogram, chest x-ray, echocardiography and cardiac catheterization can all aid in diagnosis of pericardial effusion but pericardial fluid and biopsy with histologic and cytologic analysis is required for diagnosis on underlying malignancy. Prognosis for patients with malignant pericardial effusion is primarily dictated by the underlying disease. Since outcome is usually poor, goal of treatment is palliation of symptoms and prevention of recurrence of effusion. Pericardiocentesis is useful for prevention and treatment of cardiac tamponade but inadequate in itself because of a high rate of recurrence even when followed by extended tube drainage.

Pericardial sclerosis has good success rate but high rate of complications such as arrhythmias and pericardial constriction. This makes it less preferred option than pericardial drainage; however, it may be useful for those, who are unfit for any surgical intervention. Cisplatin and tetracycline are most widely used sclerosing agents. Confirmed malignant pericardial effusion can be treated with relatively high doses of intrapericardial chemotherapy with minimal systemic side effects but the disease is restricted to only pericardium on a rare occasion. In disseminated malignancy, intrapericardial chemotherapy can improve symptoms of a hemodynamically significant effusion but other more effective and inexpensive treatment modalities may also be available.

Surgical treatment appears to result in better clinical outcome but selection of healthier patients may be confounding the results. Pericardial fenestration is the most commonly performed surgical procedure that employs subxiphoid, video-assisted thoracic surgery (VATS) and mini-thoracotomy approaches. This has an overall success rate of 93%, recurrence rate of 6% and perioperative complication rate of 4%. Subxiphoid approach can be performed under local anesthesia and does not require single-lung ventilation procedure unlike during VATS. Pericardiectomy is performed using VATS and is the second most commonly performed surgical procedure with almost 100% success rate but with a perioperative complication rate of up to 10%. Pericardio-peritoneal shunt as a treatment of malignant pericardial effusion has been reported as a safe and effective treatment but the small study population mandates further confirmatory studies. Percutaneous balloon pericardiotomy has good outcome, can be performed under local anesthesia and allows early discharge. It is useful in poor surgical candidates but has higher complications (up to 32%), which include a risk of pleural effusion, fever and pneumothorax. Outcomes tend to be better in the high-volume centers.

In conclusion, there is a paucity of high-quality studies and a lack of therapeutic options with significant impact on survival of patients with malignant pericardial effusion. Safe, cost effective and durable palliative treatment as well as treatment strategies that can prolong survival meaningfully are needed.

Chapter 5 – Cardiac tamponade is a life-threatening emergency associated with a variety of medical and surgical conditions. Since the signs and symptoms of an underlying disease are often co-manifesting, diagnosing cardiac tamponade is difficult. It is well known that cardiac tamponade patients experience mood alterations or disturbances prior to hemodynamic deterioration. Mood alterations such as being "anxious" and "restless" have been described most frequently in nursing and medical literature. A chart review study found that patients were most frequently observed as having "aggressive body movements" followed by "gets up/tries to get up" and "restless." Various kinds of facial expressions were also recorded. A short interview study of patients who had recently survived cardiac tamponade revealed that patients felt something really bad was happening, felt anxious, and couldn't stay still. Knowing characteristics of such changes in the patient's mood may help clinicians suspect cardiac tamponade. Identifying characteristic mood disturbances may facilitate further exploration of the diagnostic process including echocardiogram and may lead to timely treatment and enhanced survival.

In: Cardiac Tamponade
Editor: Cameron L. Pittman
ISBN: 978-1-63482-787-4

Chapter 1

Cardiac Tamponade: Pathophysiology, Etiology, Clinical Features, Diagnosis, and Management

Mukul Bhattarai, MD[1], Bashar Amr, MD[1], Alan Deckard, MD[1], and Mahendra K. Nepal, MD[2]
[1]Department of General Internal Medicine, Southern Illinois University, School of Medicine, Springfield, IL,US
[2]Professor, Clinical Director and Consultant Psychiatrist, Tamworth Rural Referral Hospital, Hunter New England Local Health District, Tamworth, NSW, Australia

Abstract

Cardiac tamponade is a life threatening pericardial disease which is characterized by increased pressure around the heart due to fluid accumulation in pericardial space which results in decrease in cardiac output. This condition is a medical emergency, and the complications of which include pulmonary edema, shock, and death. It is characterized by tachycardia, elevated jugular venous pressure, pulsus paradoxus, and hypotension etc. Electrocardiogram, Chest x ray and transthoracic echocardiogram are the key investigations that need to be done urgently to evaluate this clinical condition. Echocardiographically-guided percutaneous pericardiocentesis is the lifesaving procedure. Meanwhile, open surgical approach is also considered for traumatic cases, purulent pericarditis and recurrent malignant pericardial effusions. The overall mortality risk depends on the speed of diagnosis, treatment and the underlying cause of the tamponade.

In this chapter, we will review the present knowledge of the etiology, pathophysiology, diagnosis and the management of cardiac tamponade.

Introduction

Pericardial diseases and their associated hemodynamic findings have fascinated physicians for hundreds of years. Because of proximity to the vital organs like heart and lungs, these conditions are of immense clinical significance but at the same time are equally challenging in cardiovascular physiology and pathology. By definition, cardiac tamponade is a life threatening pericardial disease which is characterized by obstruction of inflow of blood to the ventricles leading to decrease of cardiac output a result of the pressure around the heart caused by accumulation of fluid within the pericardial space in a sufficient quantity. *Any large amount of pus, blood, serous fluid, loose clots, or rarely gas may accumulate and can cause cardiac tamponade.* It is suspected clinically on the grounds of presence of tachycardia, elevated jugular venous pressure, pulsus paradoxus, and hypotension etc. This condition is a medical emergency, and the complications of which include pulmonary edema, shock, and death. In this chapter we will review key elements of the anatomy and physiology of the pericardium, discuss the pathophysiology, etiology, clinical features, diagnosis, and management of cardiac tamponade.

Anatomy and Physiology of Pericardium

Before we discuss the clinical aspect of CT, we review the anatomy and physiology of the heart, specifically focusing on the pericardium.

Pericardial Layers

The heart is enclosed in a double layered fibroserous sac called the pericardium. It covers the heart and the proximal ends of the large blood vessels to which it attaches. As shown in above Figure2a, 2b, 2c, the fibrous pericardium is the outer fibrous layer of the pericardium which is the outermost tough protective cardiac tissue layer that prevents overstretching of the heart.

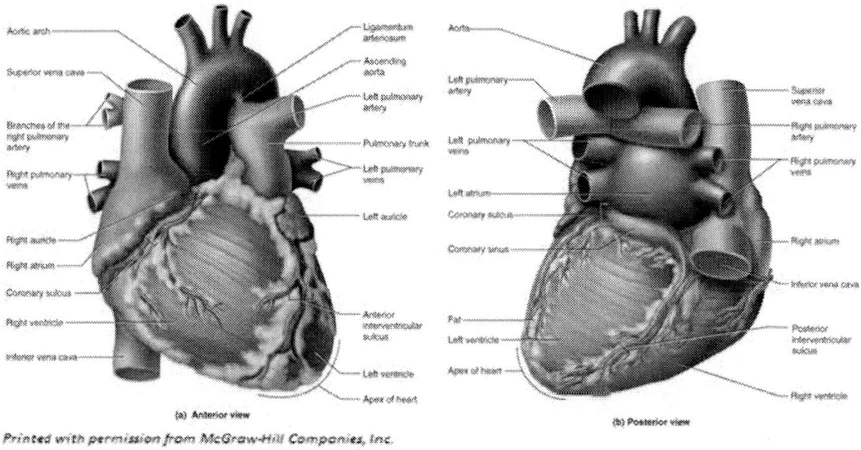

Figure 1. Exterior of heart (a) anterior (b) posterior seen after removing of pericardium.

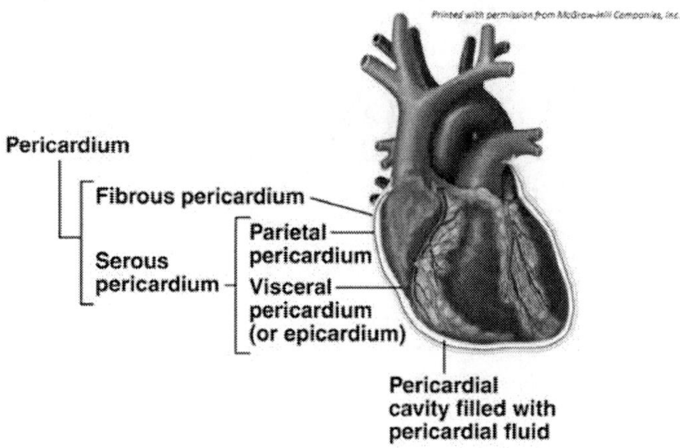

Figure 2a. Anatomy and Components of the Pericardium.

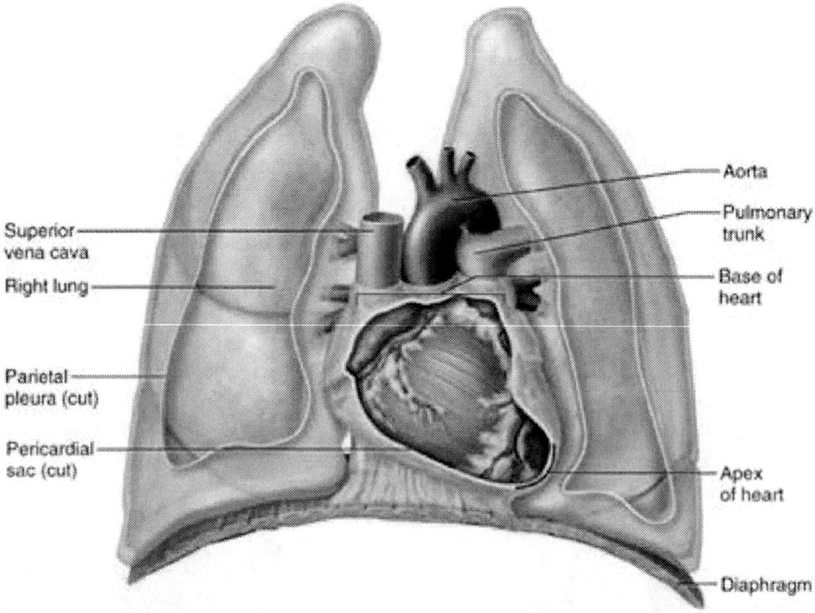

Figure 2b. Position of the Heart and Pericardium in relation to Lungs, Pleura, and Great Vessels.

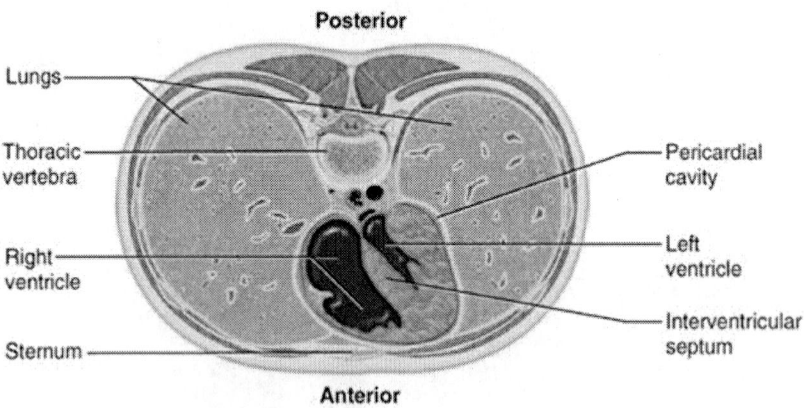

Figure 2c. Cross-sectional view of the Heart and Pericardium.

The serous layer constitutes a) visceral pericardium which is an inner serous membrane attached to the surface of the heart and b) parietal pericardium which is an outer serous membrane that lines the fibrous layer of the pericardium. The visceral pericardium, also known as epicardium, is composed of a single layer of mesothelial cells and covers both, coronary arteries and epicardial fat.

The visceral pericardium extends beyond the heart and covers about 3 cm into the root of the great vessels and reflects back upon itself to become the serous parietal pericardium, which lines the fibrous pericardium. The parietal pericardium is a fibrous structure less than 2 mm thick and predominantly composed of collagen with a lesser amount of elastin.

Pericardial Space and Pericardial Fluid

Between the visceral pericardium and the parietal pericardium of the serous layer lies the pericardial space, which normally contains 15-50 ml of fluid. This fluid lubricates the heart during each beat allowing it for friction-free motion within the pericardial space between the visceral layer of the pericardium and the outer parietal layer. The pericardium is attached to the sternum, diaphragm, and the anterior mediastinum and is invested around the great vessels and the vena cava, anchoring the heart in the thoracic cavity.

Little is known about the formation and removal of pericardial fluid, because of the paucity of comprehensive studies, especially in human subjects, and methodological difficulties to distinguish between the dynamics of normal pericardial fluid and those of a pathological effusion.

Lymphatic drainage of the pericardium to the mediastinal and tracheobronchial lymph nodes and interactions with pleural lymphatics provide the anatomical basis for pathological involvement of the pericardium in specific diseases (i.e. pleuro-pulmonary diseases such as pulmonary tuberculosis, lung cancer).

Physiology of Pericardium and Pericardial Fluid

The pericardium serves important physiologic functions. It stabilizes the heart in the chest and prevents excessive torsion while permitting the heart to beat smoothly in a friction-free compartment. The pericardial sac acts as a protective anatomical barrier preventing the spread of infection from nearby structures, specifically the lung and pleural cavities.

The pericardium is well innervated with mechanoreceptors, chemo-receptors, and phrenic afferent receptors. This innervation allows it to take part in vagally mediated reflexes (i.e. Bezold-Jarisch reflex) and produce pain with pericardial inflammation. The visceral mesothelial cells are capable of modulating structure, function, and gene expression of myocyte. The pericardium also secretes prostaglandins and substances that may modulate neural interchange and coronary tone.

Interestingly, the level of brain natriuretic peptide in the pericardial fluid is a more sensitive and accurate indicator of ventricular volume and pressure than is either plasma brain natriuretic peptide or atrial natriuretic factor, indicating it may provide the autocrine/paracrine role in heart failure. The pericardial cavity may be used as a vehicle for drug delivery and gene therapy. Studies have revealed that substances are more consistently and reproducibly able to gain access to the coronary arteries via pericardial fluid administration than endoluminal delivery.

In normal physiological conditions the intrapericardial pressure is equal to intrathoracic pressure, and it varies between +5 and -5 mm Hg during expiration and inspiration respectively. The low pressure in the pericardial cavity permits the respiratory variation in intrathoracic pressures to be mirrored in the intracardiac pressures.

Thus during *inspiration,* intrathoracic pressure decreases, causing an *increased flow into the right side* of the heart. With inspiration, there is also a decrease in the gradient between the pulmonary veins and the left atrium, causing *decreased flow into the left side* of the heart. This process is reversed during expiration.

In pericardial tamponade, the normal respiratory swings in pressure become distorted due to altered cardiac filling. Variation in right and left heart inflow then exhibits the pathophysiology of exaggerated interventricular dependence, the hallmark of pericardial tamponade *(to be discussed later).*

Pathophysiology

Hemodynamics of Pericardium in terms of Chronicity of Development of Cardiac Tamponade

The pericardial space is a closed space. The normal pressure in the pericardial space is close to zero. Therefore, fluid accumulation in such restricted intrapericardial space can potentially raise the pressure surrounding the heart to the point where cardiac filling is altered.

The amount of pericardial fluid needed to impair diastolic filling of the heart depends on the *rate* of fluid accumulation and the *compliance* of the pericardium. Rapid accumulation of as little as 150mL of fluid can result in a marked increase in pericardial pressure and can severely impede cardiac output, whereas 1000 mL of fluid may accumulate over a longer period without any significant effect on diastolic filling of the heart (Figure 3). This happens because of adaptive stretching of the pericardium over time.

A times, a compliant pericardium can allow considerable fluid accumulation over a longer period without causing any hemodynamic insult, e.g., in tuberculosis, where very large effusions can be accommodated without tamponade physiology.

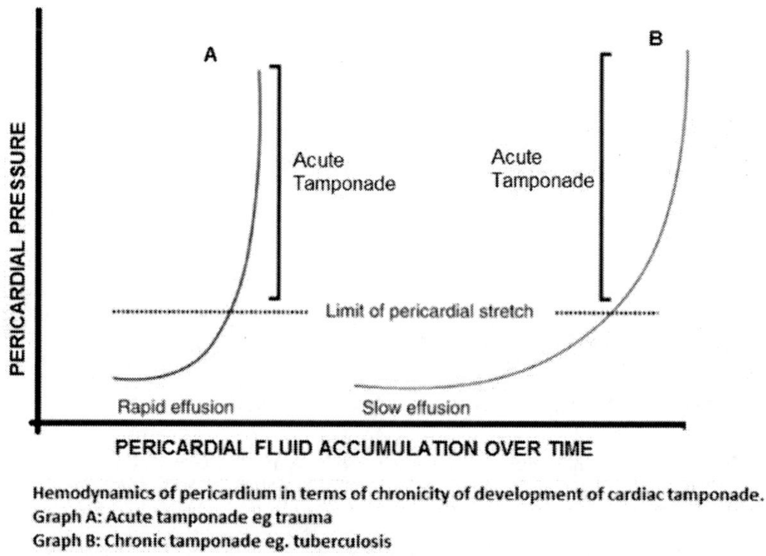

Figure 3. Pressure–volume (or strain–stress) curves depicting scenarios of volume increasing slowly or rapidly over time.

In **graph A**, rapidly increasing pericardial fluid first reaches the limit of the pericardial reserve volume (the initial flat segment) and then quickly exceeds the limit of parietal pericardial stretch, causing a steep rise in pressure, which becomes even steeper as smaller increments in fluid cause a disproportionate increase in the pericardial pressure.

Therefore, clinicians should know the tamponade physiology because it can develop before there is any evidence of large pericardial effusion.

In **graph B**, a slower rate of pericardial filling takes longer to exceed the limit of pericardial stretch, because there is more time for the pericardium to stretch and for compensatory mechanisms to become activated.

Mechanism of Development of Shock

Any increase in the intrapericardial pressure has three potential adverse effects on the heart:

(1) Limited diastolic filling from a direct compressive effect and from decreased venous return.
(2) Increased diastolic filling pressures.
(3) Reduced stroke volume and cardiac output.

CLINICAL PEARL 1
Clinical Signs in Tamponade Based on Pathophysiology

Increase intrapericardial pressure, compression of heart chambers, decrease venous return → decrease CO

Diastolic pressures increase and equalize in all cardiac chambers→ minimal flow of blood from RA to RV when TV opens→ blunted Y descent

Increase ventricular interdependence →pulsus paradoxus

Inspiration → increase intrapericardial & RA pressures→ increase venous return → increase RV size → septal shift to left, Also, Increase pulmonary vascular compliance→ decrease venous return. Result is decrease LV filling → decrease LV, stroke volume and blood pressure.

Right heart has lower pressures and thinner wall. Therefore, it is most vulnerable to compression early by a pericardial effusion, and ***abnormal right heart filling is the earliest sign*** of a hemodynamically significant pericardial effusion.

RA: right atrium, RV: right ventricle, TB: tricuspid valve

When intrapericardial pressure becomes higher than intracavitary pressure, compression of the heart occurs with reduced diastolic filling. This is first seen on the right side, rather than the left, due to the thinner walls and reduced chamber pressure. Therefore, the *right atrium is usually compressed before the right ventricle and abnormal right heart filling is the earliest sign of a hemodynamically significant pericardial effusion.* Under these conditions, adequate filling of the right heart requires a compensatory increase in systemic venous pressure, achieved from venoconstriction and fluid retention. If diastolic compression becomes too significant to be overcome by elevated filling pressures and other compensatory mechanisms, cardiac output and blood pressure will fall. Systemic venous pressure is impaired throughout the cardiac cycle in cardiac tamponade, resulting in right atrial and right ventricular collapse. Because the pulmonary vascular bed is a vast and compliant circuit, blood preferentially accumulates in the venous circulation, at the expense of left ventricular filling. This results in reduced cardiac output and venous return.

Systemic Venous Return in Cardiac Tamponade

To understand the relation between venous and pericardial pressures in cardiac tamponade, it is useful to review the normal biphasic pattern of venous return.

The first wave of venous return occurs at the onset of ventricular ejection, and is accompanied by a small reduction in intrapericardial pressure. A second surge of venous return occurs in early diastole, when the tricuspid valve opens and atrial pressure decreases.

In *cardiac tamponade, venous return is unimodal and is confined to ventricular systole.* As the spectrum of cardiac tamponade progresses, venous return is impaired in diastole, at a time when cardiac volume and intrapericardial pressure are maximal. Since the inspiratory fall in intrathoracic pressure is transmitted to the pericardial space, the normal inspiratory increase in systemic venous return is preserved.

This reflection of respiratory variation on venous return and cardiac output is exaggerated in cardiac tamponade and is one key component of development of pulsus paradoxus, as discussed later in the chapter.

Ventricular Interdependance

Ventricular interdependence is an important phenomenon which occurs as a result of reciprocal respiratory variation in volume of blood flow in right and left heart across atrioventricular valves.

The amount of blood flow into one ventricle is dependent on the amount of blood flow into the other ventricle, and is directly associated with respiratory mechanics of each person.

- **During inspiration,** the negative intra-thoracic pressure is transmitted to the cardiac chambers, creating a depression in the right ventricle and atrium which suctions the vena caval flow into the right atrium. The *right ventricle expands while the left ventricle volume decreases* as a result of septal shift to left. Meanwhile, the increase in pulmonary vascular compliance results in a decrease in venous return to left side of heart.
- **During expiration,** the pressures in the thorax and in the pericardium are summed and are superior to the pressure in the right chambers, and thus the right ventricle is compressed. When the space is filled by an effusion, the cardiac chambers become smaller. Diastolic expansion is limited and interventricular dependence is increased because the pericardium cannot be stretched. These factors lead to further *right ventricular compression.*

This consequence of exaggerated ventricular interdependence in cardiac tamponade can be assessed from parasternal long or short axis viewing both right and left ventricles as shown (Figure 4 and Figure 5).

Normal pericardial space transmits respiratory variation in thoracic pressure to the heart. As a result, any increase in pericardial pressure such as in cardiac tamponade intensifies the interdependence of the cardiac chambers when the total cardiac volume is limited by the large pericardial effusion.

The volume in any cardiac chamber can only increase when there is an equal decrease in the volume in other chambers. Thus, venous return and atrial filling predominantly occur during ventricular systole as the ejection of blood out of the right and left ventricles lowers cardiac volume and allows blood to enter the atria.

Moreover, the normal effects of respiration are accentuated such that venous return and right-sided filling occur during inspiration as intrathoracic pressures fall, providing a pressure gradient from the systemic veins to the right atrium. This small normal respiratory variation in left ventricular stroke volume and systolic arterial pressure is markedly accentuated in cardiac tamponade, resulting in the clinical finding of "paradoxical pulse" (discussed later).

Inflow of blood accross AV valves during inspiration and expiration:

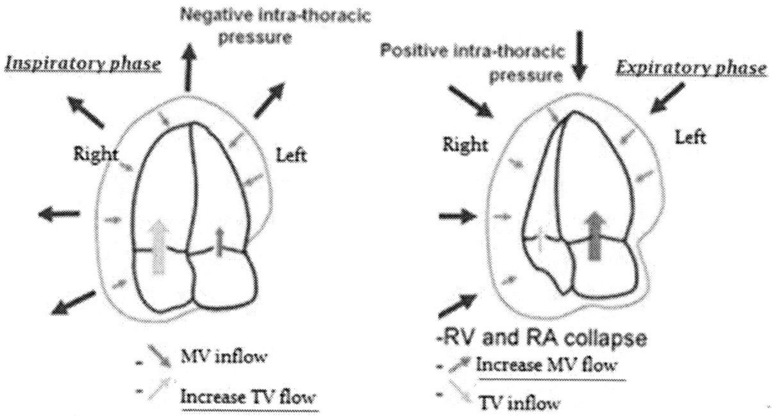

Modified:
From https://web.stanford.edu/group/ccm_echocardio/cgi-bin/mediawiki/index.php/Tamponade

Figure 4. Exaggerated interventricular interdependence is classic feature of cardiac tamponade even though there is variable degree of compression of the heart occurring during all parts of cardiac cycle. *Normally systemic venous return to the right heart increases with inspiration, and pulmonary venous return to the left heart decreases with inspiration producing some interventricular interdependence as shown.* AV valves: atrioventricular valve, RV: right ventricle, RA: right atrium, TV: tricuspid valve, MV: mitral valve.

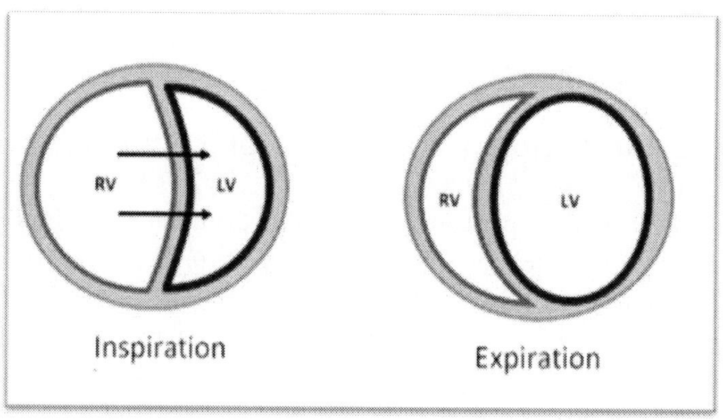

Figure 5. Schematic diagram showing exaggerated ventricular interdependence. In cardiac tamponade, systemic venous return increases with inspiration enlarging the right side of the heart and encroaching on the left (shown by two black arrows). Just opposite happens with expiration: right ventricle is compressed.

Because the total intrapericardial volume is fixed by the pressurized effusion, this increased inspiratory right ventricular filling impairs the filling of left ventricle. *Thus left heart filling occurs predominantly during expiration when there is less filling of the right heart.*

Transmural Pressures in Cardiac Tamponade

Another way of comprehending the progression of reduced venous filling in cardiac tamponade is through the understanding of the transmural pressures. The *transmural pressure of each cardiac chamber, defined as intracardiac pressure minus pericardial pressure*, is a key determinant of its filling. It is considered a true filling (distending) pressure that contributes to ventricular preload.

Pericardial pressure is usually zero and fluctuates with respect to intrathoracic pressure. In a normal patient the pericardial pressure is lower than right mean atrial and right ventricular diastolic pressure, thus right atrial transmural filling pressure is higher than its cavitary pressure. *In tamponade, rising pericardial pressure progressively reduces the average transmural pressure of the right and subsequently the left cardiac chambers.*

For example, if an accumulating pericardial effusion elevates pericardial pressure to 15 mmHg and right atrial pressure (measured or estimated from JVP) is 17 mmHg, the transmural filling pressure is only 2 mmHg, indicating a hypovolemic state and poor venous filling of the cardiac chamber despite elevated neck veins.

Equalization of Diastolic Pressure throughout the Heart

As mentioned earlier, pericardial pressure is distributed equally among all chambers of heart because of free flowing nature of pericardial fluid. This reduces the gradients between chambers throughout diastole which is usually not evident with small effusions, but becomes hemodynamically significant in large effusions whereby greater pressure in the pericardium is transmitted to all four cardiac chambers causing an "*equalization of central pressures*".

The reduction of the pressure gradient between the atria and the ventricles when the AV valves open means that there is less transfer of blood from the atria to the ventricles. This phenomenon of equalization of diastolic pressure is often discussed with cardiac tamponade pathophysiology. It is perceived as a loss of the y-descent of the CVP or PCWP waveform tracings.

The clinical conditions where equalization of pressure occur will be elaborated later.

Changes in Neck Vein Waves

Before discussing the pathophysiological changes in neck vein waves in cardiac tamponade, we will briefly discuss the mechanism of development of different neck vein waves in normal person.

Pressure changes in right atrium are reflected in jugular venous pulse. The atrial waveforms are composed of three positive waves, the A, C, and V waves, and two negative waves, the X and Y descents (Figure 6a).

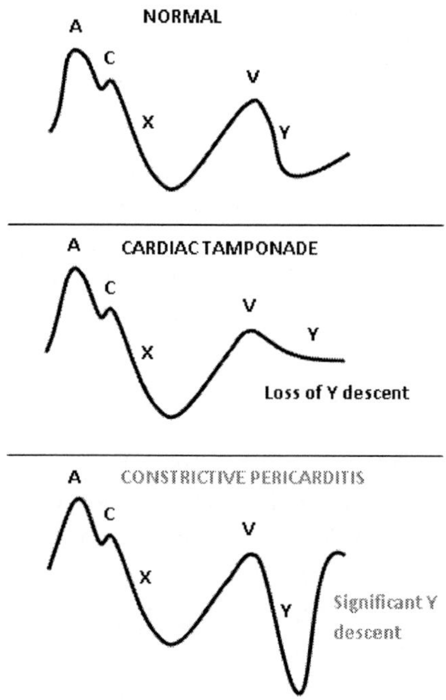

6a: Normal jugular venous wave.

6b: Jugular venous wave in cardiac tamponade showing loss of Y descent.

6c: Jugular venous wave in constrictive pericarditis showing significant Y descent.

Figure 6. Jugular venous wave in different clinical conditions.

The **A wave** is a result of atrial systole, and both the rapidity and amplitude of the A wave upstroke are a reflection of the strength of atrial contraction.

The ensuing **C wave** represents tricuspid valve displacement toward the right atrium during early ventricular systole. The C wave is not normally seen on physical examination, and if noticed should indicate tricuspid valve pathology.

These positive waves are followed by the **X descent**, which is associated with decline in intrapericardial pressure. This decline in pressure is due to atrial relaxation, movement of the tricuspid apparatus toward the ventricular apex, and pericardial emptying during ventricular systole.

During late ventricular systole, there is an increase in the right atrial pressure due to the filling of the right atrium against a closed tricuspid valve. This represents the positive **V wave**.

The subsequent **Y descent** coincides with the opening of the atrioventricular valves, early ventricular diastole, and atrial emptying and depressurization.

CLINICAL PEARL 2 **Neck Vein Waves in Cardiac Tamponade**
Y descent is lost because there is no systemic venous return to ventricle during early diastole due to elevated pericardiac pressure. **X descent is retained, which is represented as venous inflow after blood ejection during ventricular systole.**

In cardiac tamponade, the hallmark jugular venous pressure waveform abnormality is the *loss of the Y descent*. This is due to the concept that in severe tamponade the total heart volume is fixed. The right atrium and right ventricle develop equalization in pressure in cardiac tamponade, causing *a lack of flow across the tricuspid valve in early ventricular diastole*. Therefore, blood can enter the heart only when blood is simultaneously leaving, at the time of ventricular systole corresponding to the X descent.

In other words, in cardiac tamponade there is fixed cardiac volumes, *no systemic venous return during early diastole, and no Y descent.* The X descent is retained because it occurs during ventricular systole when the blood leaving from the heart momentarily provides some pressure relief (Figure 6b).

Classification and Etiology

There are many causes of cardiac tamponade. The majority of literature suggests that any cause of pericarditis can be responsible for development of pericardial effusion followed and cardiac tamponade (Table 2, 3).

Table 1. Classification of Pericardial Effusion

Onset
- Acute (> 1 week)
- Subacute (1 week - 3 months)
- Chronic (> 3 months)

Size
- Mild (<10 mm)
- Moderate (10–20 mm)
- Large (>20 mm)

Distribution
- Circumferential
- Loculated

Hemodynamic effect
- Without cardiac tamponade
- With cardiac tamponade
- Effusive-constrictive

Composition/type
- Transudate
- Exudate
- Hydropericardium (transudate, plasma ultrafiltrate)
- Hemopericardium (blood in pericardial space)
- Chylopericardium (chylous pericardial fluid)
- Pyopericardium (purulent pericardial effusion)
- Pneumopericardium (air in the pericardium)

No precise definition is available for acute and subacute pericardial effusion, while the definition of chronic as >3 months is more clearly defined.

European Heart Journal (2013) 34, 1186–1197 doi:10.1093/eurheartj/ehs372

Therefore, before discussing the specific etiologies of cardiac tamponade, it is important to know about the classification (Table 1) and etiologies of pericardial effusion since it may guide the clinician to the presence or absence of pericardial tamponade in the setting of underlying pathology.

Large idiopathic chronic effusion (>3 months) have a 30-35% risk of progression to cardiac tamponade. Subacute (4 to 6 weeks) large effusions not responsive to conventional therapy and with echocardiographic signs of right chamber collapse may have an increased risk of progression to cardiac tamponade. Preventive drainage is recommended in such cases.

Table 2. Among etiologies for tamponade, *Merce et al* reported the following incidence rates

- Malignant diseases - 30-60% of cases
- Uremia - 10-15% of cases
- Idiopathic pericarditis - 5-15%
- Infectious diseases - 5-10%
- Anticoagulation - 5-10%
- Connective tissue diseases - 2-6%
- Dressler or postpericardiotomy syndrome - 1-2%

***PerCornily et al (2008): Malignant disease was the primary cause of medical tamponade (74 patients; 65%), followed by viral history (11; 10%) and intra-pericardial bleeding due to anti-coagulation treatment (4; 3%). In 12 cases, etiology remained unknown.10%).

Based on the Composition of the Fluid

Cardiac tamponade can be classified as serous, serosanguineous, hemorrhagic, or chylous etc.

Based on chronicity of underlying etiology: It can be acute, subacute, or chronic:

1. **Acute tamponade:**
   It usually occurs due to traumatic rupture of ventricle as a result of a procedure or blunt trauma and also in aortic dissection or myocardial infarction with ventricular rupture. Infection is the rare cause of acute tamponade. However several cases of bacterial infection causing acute purulent cardiac tamponade have been reported in literature.

2. **Subacute/chronic tamponade:**
   - Infection: More commonly bacterial than viral.
   - Malignancy: Particularly lung, breast, Hodgkin's, mesothelioma
   - Post-MI, post-CT surgery, post-procedure
   - Uremia
   - Post-chemotherapy agents
   - Collagen-vascular disease: in particular SLE
   - HIV
   - Idiopathic

Common Specific Etiologies

Malignancy

Malignant diseases as a group are the most common cause of pericardial tamponade. It accounts for 30-60% cases of cardiac tamponade. Theoretically, any malignancy can cause a pericardial effusion. Lung cancer, breast cancer, and Hodgkin's lymphoma are the most common malignancies which can cause tamponade.

Infection

Multiple infectious etiologies of pericardial effusion exist. Bacterial pericardial effusions occur as a complication of an infectious focus originating elsewhere in the body which reaches the pericardial space hematogenously or by direct spread. It rarely occurs as a primary site of infection. Therefore, *in any diagnose case of purulent tamponade; clinician should always search for the primary source of infection.* The organisms usually invade as opportunistic pathogens from the remote source through a subtle break in the mucosa and set up pericardial infection in immunocompromised patients and in other circumstances such as in surgical or other trauma or when tumors arise at the mucosal surface.

The common causes of bacterial pericarditis are gram-positive cocci, mostly *Staphylococcus aureus and Streptococcus pneumonia, Streptococcus viridans, and Group A Streptococcus.* Furthermore, certain gram-negative anaerobic organisms such as *Bacteroidesfragilis, Prevotella, Porphyromonas, and Fusobacterium* are discussed in the literature as causes of purulent pericarditis.

Table 3. Causes of Pericardial Disease and Precipitating Factors causing Cardiac Tamponade

Likely to progress to cardiac tamponade

- Neoplastic diseases
- Infections (i.e. viral: EBV, CMV enteroviruses, HIV, bacterial, especially tuberculosis)
- Iatrogenic hemopericardium
- Post-traumatic pericardial effusion
- Post-cardiotomy syndrome
- Hemopericardium in aortic dissection and rupture of the heart after acute myocardial infarction
- Renal failure

Rarely progressing to cardiac tamponade

- Systemic autoimmune disease
- Autoreactive pericardial effusions
- Hypo- or hyperthyreosis
- Early and late pericarditis (Dressler's syndrome) in acute myocardial infarction
- Any other aetiology of pericardial disease (i.e. cholesterol pericarditis, chylopericardium)
- Never progressing to cardiac tamponade
- Pericardial transudates caused by heart failure or pulmonary hypertension
- Pericardial transudates in the last trimester of normal pregnancy

Precipitating factors

Drugs

- Antihypertensive medications
- Anticoagulants, thrombolytics, etc.

Injury

- Complex PCI
- Pacemaker implantation
- Endomyocardial biopsy
- Recent cardiac surgery
- Indwelling instrumentation
- Blunt chest trauma

Septicemia

Dehydration, diuretics (decrease volume status)

European Heart Journal (2013) 34, 1186–1197
doi:10.1093/eurheartj/ehs372

The other rare anaerobes isolated from patients with pericarditis are *Peptostreptococcus, Clostridium, Bifidobacterium, Actinomyces species, and Propionibacterium.*

Etiologies due to polymicrobial agents are just limited to case reports.

Bacterial pericarditis with or without tamponade is associated with considerable morbidity and death despite the advances in diagnosis and is considered a life-threatening condition with a fatality rate of 100% if untreated. In addition, constrictive pericarditis occurs over the course of purulent pericarditis in at least 3.5% of the cases even after optimum management.

Fortunately, the incidence of bacterial purulent pericarditis has become rare since the advent of antibiotic usage, particularly in the developed world wherein the incidence of such pericarditis and tamponade accounts for less than 1% of pericarditis cases.

Tuberculosis has historically been the most important cause of pericardial effusion and tamponade. However, in the United States and other developed nations the incidence is decreasing to the point of being rare. Large pericardial effusions are uncommon, and manifestation as cardiac tamponade isscarce.

In a series of 231 consecutive patients with pericardial disease, 7% of cases of tamponade were related to tuberculosis, and three of nine cases of tuberculous pericarditis initially manifested as tamponade. It continues to be one of the most important etiologies, mainly among the populations of Asian and African origin. Nowadays, most cases of tuberculous cardiac tamponade are seen in patients with AIDS. A pericardial effusion from tuberculosis can occur in isolation in the absence of any other pulmonary manifestations. Since the diagnosis of tuberculosis may be delayed due to the slow-growing nature of the bacterium, clinicians need to be aware of this possibility and consider the use of modern diagnostic techniques that may permit an earlier diagnosis of tuberculosis.

A high index of clinical suspicions and a comprehensive history including demography is essential to diagnose tuberculosis effusion. It is associated with a high mortality if untreated and a high risk of evolution into constrictive pericarditis (30–50% of cases) even after optimum treatment. A previous history of tuberculosis, an origin from an area, where tuberculosis is endemic (i.e. mainly Africa and Asia), a subacute course, low grade fever, weight loss, night sweats, a moderate to large pericardial effusion are all features associated with a high risk of a tuberculous cause of the effusion.

A definitive diagnosis of tuberculous effusion/tamponade requires the demonstration of tuberculosis bacilli in pericardial fluid or tissue. However, the diagnosis is considered as probable in patients with the diagnoses of tuberculosis elsewhere in the body (i.e. pulmonary), or with a lymphocytic pericardial exudate with elevated adenosine deaminase (ADA) levels.

The empiric response to antituberculosis therapycan also help to diagnose tuberculosis in an endemic area, but not in Western Europe and North America. Multidrug-resistant (MDR) and extensively drug-resistant (XDR) TB are of particular concern among HIV-infected or other immunocompromised people.

Other infectious causes: Viral pericarditis or myocarditis can ultimately cause pericardial effusion. It is most commonly associated with Coxsackie B virus infection. Rarely, such effusion progresses to tamponade. Viral pericarditis may pave the way for a more serious bacterial pericarditis as a secondary super-imposed bacterial infection. Fungal pericardial involvement is rare.

Iatrogenic pericardial effusions are common after cardiac surgery and frequently require drainage. Radiation therapy less commonly causes pericardial effusions, especially with availability of dose reduction therapy today. For unclear reasons, minoxidil, penicillins and methysergide have been shown to cause pericardial effusion. However, tamponade physiology is uncommon after stopping the offending agents including medications.

Hemorrhage into the pericardium from trauma, aortic dissection or left ventricular free wall rupture after a myocardial infarction can occur. Hemorrhage into the pericardium or hemopericardium during invasive procedures such as percutaneous coronary intervention complicating with coronary perforation or pacemaker insertion complicating with right ventricular perforation can cause acute tamponade.

Autoimmune reactions are important causes of acute pericarditis and pericardial effusions. Common autoimmune disorders such as systemic lupus erythematosus (both primary and drug-induced- hydralazine, quinidine or isoniazid etc), rheumatoid arthritis and scleroderma can cause autoimmune pericarditis and pericardial effusions.

Dressler's syndrome is an autoimmune reaction that occurs after myocardial infarction causing pericarditis and effusion. Occasionally, idiopathic pericardial effusions are considered to be an autoimmune mediated, however the etiology remains unclear.

Metabolic causes of a pericardial effusion include **hypothyroidism** and **uremia,** and are a result from increased capillary permeability in these disease states. Uremia accounts for 10-15% of cases of tamponade.

Organ failure in the form of **congestive heart failure, liver failure, and renal failure** may all cause pericardial effusion. In the setting of heart failure there is an increased hydrostatic pressure leading to a development of an effusion. On the other hand, pericardial fluid accumulation in liver and renal failure results due to decreased oncotic pressure.

Transmural myocardial infarctions can sometimes infarct the pericardium as well causing an inflammatory reaction, pericarditis, and a pericardial effusion.

Rare cause of tamponade physiology: External compression of the pericardial sac can cause tamponade physiology such as in large pleural effusions.

CLINICAL PEARL 3

Beck's Triad:

First described in 1935, are characterized as

- Hypotension
- Jugular venous distention
- Muffled heart sounds

Present only in present 10% to 40% of tamponade cases.

Other Clinical Features of Cardiac Tamponade:

- Tachycardia/Tachypnea
- Pulsus Paradoxus
- Diaphoresis
- Narrow pulse pressure
- Peripheral Cyanosis
- Symptoms/Signs of Underlying Etiology
- Chest Pain, atypical chest discomfort
- Palpitation

Idiopathic: Despite advancements in technology, the etiology may not be found in a large number of tamponade cases. It is recommended that underlying causes be aggressively sought in all cases in order to provide the appropriate treatment and prevent recurrence.

Clinical Features

The clinical features of cardiac tamponade depend mainly on the size of the effusion and the underlying etiology. Nevertheless, any patient with dyspnea, elevated jugular venous pressure (JVP), low blood pressure, and edema (or any combination of these symptoms) a diagnosis of cardiac tamponade should be considered.

Beck's triad, consisting of hypotension, jugular venous distension and muffled heart sounds are characteristic features of cardiac tamponade. It present in only 10-40% of cases.

Cardiac tamponade should be considered in the differential diagnosis of any patients with shock or pulseless electric activity as well. The clinical presentations depend on chronicity of fluid accumulation in the pericardial space. *Patients may just present with hemodynamic instability if pericardial fluid accumulates rapidly, even in small amounts, as discussed in pathophysiology* (Figure #3). *Sometimes, patients may present with chronic dyspnea, and have a large effusion with tamponade physiology on investigation.* The classical features of tamponade are usually associated with circumferential effusions. Loculated effusion can be difficult to diagnose because it can cause focal tamponade.

Pulsus paradoxus

Another hallmark of cardiac tamponade beside Beck's triad is **pulsus paradoxus**. **Pulsus paradoxus** or **pathological paradoxical pulse** is defined as *an inspiratory decrease in systolic blood pressure greater than 10 mmHg.* Before discussing the pathophysiology of pulsus paradoxus in the setting of cardiac tamponade, we will review on normal physiology behind the paradoxical pulse.

Normally, the effects of respiratory oscillations on the right and the left heart are dissimilar due to the differences in the anatomic relationships of the respective venous return systems to the intrapleural space. Though both right heart chambers are intrathoracic, the tributary systemic venous system is extrapleural.

Normal inspiration causes a decrease in intrathoracic pressure (ITP), which in turn enhances the filling gradient from the extrathoracic systemic veins to the right atrium. This pressure difference between systemic veins and right atrium (filling gradient) augments venous return flow by 50-60%, and increases right heart filling and output.

CLINICAL PEARL 4 **Pathological Paradoxical Pulse:**
• >10-mm Hg drop in systolic arterial pressure during inspiration. • It's sensitivity is 82%, specificity is 70% *(JAMA2007)*

CLINICAL PEARL 5 **Causes of Pulsus Paradoxus:**
• Cardiac Tamponade • Severe COPD • Pulmonary Embolism (approximately 30% of the time) • Constrictive Pericarditis • Restrictive Cardiomyopathy • Hemorrhagic/Hypovolemic shock • Marked Obesity • Partial Obstruction of the Superior Vena Cava

On the other hand, the left heart chambers and its tributary pulmonary veins are entirely intrathoracic. Thus, pleural pressure changes are evenly distributed and there is minimal change in the pressure gradient from the pulmonary veins to the left heart with respiration. As a result both early diastolic transmitral filling pressure and left ventricular filling are essentially unchanged throughout the respiratory cycle. However, the left heart filling, stroke volume, and aortic systolic pressure normally decrease with inspiration up to the pressure of 10 mmHg.

A number of mechanisms are responsible for this normal inspiratory oscillation in aortic pressure, including ventricular competition for intrapericardial volume related to leftward septal displacement induced by augmented right heart filling (ventricular interdependence), increased left ventricular afterload imposed by the differential effects of decrease ITP on the heart relative to the extra thoracic great vessels, and inspiratory delay of augmented right ventricular output through the lungs.

Pulsus paradoxus or pathological paradoxical pulse is a characteristic finding in patients with cardiac tamponade, and is an ominous sign of hemodynamic compromise. As the pericardium becomes more crowded and intrapericardial space becomes more limited, the increasing intrapericadial pressure accentuates the coupling of the ventricles. Under these conditions, increased filling on one side of the heart results in a concomitant decrement in filling on the contralateral chamber.

In patients with hemodynamically significant effusions, the intracardiac and systemic venous pressures are markedly elevated but inspiratory augmentation of venous return is intact and is a major mechanism for pulsus paradoxus. As inspiratory preload of the right heart competes for space in the crowded high pressure pericardium, it compresses the left heart through ventricular interaction across the septum.

In tamponade physiology the respiratory variation in pulmonary wedge pressure is greater than that of the intrapericardial pressure. Thus with inspiration, there is a reduced pulmonary wedge to pericardial pressure gradient. In severe cardiac tamponade pericardial pressure approximates to left ventricular diastolic pressure. Therefore inspiration results in a larger decrement in wedge pressure as compared to left ventricular pressure, reducing the gradient for left ventricular filling, decreasing mitral valve flow, and decreasing left ventricular filling.

Overall inspiration in the setting of severe tamponade results in reduced left ventricular preload, stroke volume, and cardiac output manifesting as pulsus paradoxus. This can be measured as a drop in aortic systolic blood pressure greater than 10 mmHg, or *in hemodynamically end-stage tamponade the paradoxical pulse may manifest as an absence of a palpable brachial or radial pulse during inspiration.*

A paradoxical pulse is not pathognomic of tamponade, and its specificity is only 70%, as it can also occur in other conditions when there are wide swings in intrathoracic pressure usually in the setting of respiratory distress such as pulmonary embolism, hypovolemic shock, severe COPD, constriction and right ventricular infarct etc.

It is important to understand that the paradoxical pulse may be difficult to recognize in the presence of severe shock, and may be absent in cardiac tamponade if there is coexisting aortic insufficiency, atrial septal defect, or preexisting elevated left ventricular end-diastolic pressure due to left ventricular hypertrophy or dilatation, pulmonary hypertension.

How to Measure Paradoxical Pulse

1. Slowly deflate the cuff until you start hearing any Korotkoffs ounds. At the highest blood pressure when you **hear Korotkoff sounds intermittently** (rather than with every heart beat), note the blood pressure. (This first sound will only be heard **during expiration**.).
2. Continue to lower the cuff pressure to the highest value at which you **hear Korotkoff sounds with each beat**; this means that you are hearing sounds with **inspiration and expiration.**
3. The difference between #1 and #2 is the "pulsus paradoxus." If it is more than 10 mmHg, it is considered significant.
4. Remember, in normal person, systolic blood pressure (SBP) can drop upto 10-mm Hg during inspiration. Therefore, paradoxical pulse is an exaggeration of normal physiology.

Note: You can even test pulsus paradoxus on yourself by feeling your radial pulse during a deep inspiration. There is a subtle, but definite decrease in the amplitude of the pulsation.

Differential Diagnosis

The differential diagnosis of cardiac tamponade is broad. It usually depends on severity of presentation:

1. **Acute cardiac tamponade**: acute myocardial infarction (especially with right ventricular involvement, typically present as elevated JVP and hypotension), significant pulmonary embolism, and an aortic dissection.

   Acute myocardial infarction is associated with characteristic electrocardiographic changes of infarction and the latter, in the absence of cardiac tamponade, should not cause an increase in JVP.
2. **Subacute cardiac tamponade**, in which patients typically present with dyspnea, fatigue, elevated JVP, and edema, must also be distinguished from *constrictive pericarditis, congestive heart failure, and advanced liver disease with cirrhosis*. Echocardiography is critically important in making this distinction, as it may identify other

cardiac pathology consistent with congestive heart failure or constrictive pericarditis.

In addition, patients with cirrhosis typically have jaundice and abnormalities of hepatic synthetic function (e.g., elevated prothrombin time). A large pleural effusion can also produce signs of cardiac tamponade that resolve after thoracentesis.

Constrictive Pericarditis

Constrictive pericarditis is an important cause of *diastolic dysfunction* or diastolic heart failure and can present in a similar way: dyspnea, elevated JVP, tachycardia etc. This condition is widely discussed as the *one of the most common differential diagnosis of Cardiac tamponade*. The diastolic filling pattern during each cardiac cycle and the response to respiration differ in constrictive pericarditis and tamponade. The distinctive hemodynamic profiles are recognized.

Similarities and differences in hemodynamic profile in Cardiac tamponade and Constrictive pericarditis: (Table 4).

First, cardiac tamponade causes continuous compression of the heart throughout the cardiac cycle. The ventricles are compressed at end-systole and early diastole. This prevents rapid atrial emptying and rapid ventricular filling in early diastole, for this reason, the right atrial waveform shows attenuation or loss of the diastolic Y descent, as illustrated in Figure 6, whereas in constrictive pericarditis the early diastolic ventricular filling is explosively rapid and abruptly abbreviated. The right ventricular waveform shows elevation of diastolic pressure throughout diastole and the absence of the dip-and-plateau pattern in cardiac tamponade. Because stroke volume is depressed, right ventricular pulse pressure is reduced and right ventricular and pulmonary artery systolic pressures are normal or reduced. This happens because the pericardial cavity is obliterated and the pericardium does not transmit these pressure changes. The dissociation of intrathoracic and intracardiac pressures along with ventricular interaction is the basis for the physical, hemodynamic and echocardiographic findings of constriction.

The *thickened pericardium in constrictive pericarditis does not restrict chamber enlargement at low volumes* and therefore *does not impair early diastolic filling* but at higher volumes the limiting constraint is reached and filling is limited and the pressures in all chambers will become equal. *Filling is preserved in early diastole* resulting in persistent of y descent as shown in Figure 6 but compromised in late diastole.

The symmetric surface pressure of the constricting pericardium usually impairs diastolic filling and increase the diastolic pressures of all chambers of the heart. Right and left ventricular diastolic pressures are and usually equal within 5 mm Hg or less. Pulmonary artery and right ventricular systolic pressures are usually between 35 and 45 mm Hg.

Pulmonary artery systolic pressure may be low (reflecting reduced right ventricular stroke volume and pulse pressure) or mildly elevated if chronic left a trial hypertension has caused a secondary increase in pulmonary vascular resistance. Severe pulmonary hypertension is not a feature of constrictive pericarditis and is indicative of coexisting heart or pulmonary disease.

CLINICAL PEARL 6 Kussmaul's Sign:
Defined as a paradoxical rise in jugular venous pressure upon inspiration. Causes Include: Constrictive Pericarditis Right Ventricular Infarction Right Ventricular failure Restrictive Cardiomyopathy Tricuspid Stenosis

In addition, both pericardial constriction and cardiac tamponade increase ventricular interdependance, in which filling of one ventricle limits simultaneous filling of the other, which is mediated by both the mechanical constraint of the pericardium and the shared interventricular septum.

A key contemporary model characterizes the nature of pericardial constraint in cardiac tamponade as "coupled" constraint exerted by uniform liquid pressure on the heart, versus "uncoupled" constraint exerted by regional surface pressure in pericardial constriction.

Coupled constraint (tamponade) produces greater gains in ventricular interdependence than constriction, so that severely increased inspiratory filling of the right ventricle results in highly coupled reduction in filling of the left ventricle and the occurrence of pulsus paradoxus, whereas uncoupled constraint (constriction) has a more modest effect on ventricular interdependence but greatly modifies the effective elastance of the thin-walled right ventricle. This increases the occurrence of **Kussmaul's sign**, which is the rise in jugular venous pressure with inspiration due to impaired filling of the right ventricle and the jugular veins instead become engorged.

Table 4. Key Differences between Cardiac Tamponade and Constrictive Pericarditis

	Cardiac tamponade	Constrictive pericarditis
1. Pulsus paradoxus	Usually present	Less common
2. Systemic venous wave morphology in Jugular vein	Absence Y descent	Prominent Y descent (diastolic dip)
3. Kussmaul Sign-**see text** for description	Less common	More common
4. Systemic venous return with inspiration	Increases	Does not increase with inspiration under resting conditions
5. Square root sign or dip and plateau sign in ventricular pressure during diastole	Absent	Present
6. Pericardial knock	Absent	Present
7. Early ventricular filling	Impaired	Enhanced
8. Right Atrial Collapse and RVDC	Present	Absent
9. Electrical alternans	May be present	Absent
10. Thickened/Calcified pericardium	Absent	Present

RVDC: right ventricular diastolic collapse.

Note that decreased intrathoracic pressure during inspiration normally leads to an increase in venous return to the right side of the heart causing decrease in jugular venous pressure. This paradoxical rise in jugular venous pressure upon inspiration defines **Kussmaul's sign**, and is not a feature of cardiac tamponade. Though pericardial and right atrial pressures are elevated in cardiac tamponade, both fall during inspiration.

The occurrence of pulsus paradoxus in constrictive pericarditis is variable, and depends on the presence of inspiratory variation of right and left ventricular filling and the magnitude of ventricular interdependence. This is in contrast to cardiac tamponade, in which severely exaggerated inspiratory filling of the right ventricle occurs at the expense of left ventricular filling, and pulsus paradoxus is a striking hemodynamic finding in almost all patients.

To summarize, with pericardial tamponade, the total pericardial space is constrained due to the effusion. Thus, the normal bulging of the RV into the LV is exaggerated and limits left sided filling even more. In addition, there is probably more filling and pooling of blood in the pulmonary vasculature since it is more distensible. Again, this is an exaggeration of normal physiology and systolic blood pressure declines.

The presence of a *pericardial knock* (accentuated heart sound occurring slightly earlier than a third heart sound due to abrupt cessation of early diastolic filling) favors constrictive pericarditis.

Table 5. Clinical Conditions of Equalization of Ventricular Diastolic Pressures *(Chatterjee K Circulation: Heart Failure. 2011; 4: 374-377)*

Acute	Chronic
Cardiac tamponade	Restrictive cardiomyopathy
Right ventricular myocardial infarction	Constrictive pericarditis
Pulmonary embolism	Severe tricuspid regurgitation
	Dilated LV failure with primary or secondary RV failure
	Left-sided heart failure with preserved ejection fraction complicated by secondary RV failure

LV: left ventricle, RV: right ventricle.

Pericardial imaging, cardiac catheterization and even pericardial biopsy will be required to differentiate the constrictive pericarditis from restrictive cardiomyopathy. Pericardial imaging may show increased thickness or calcification of the pericardium favoring the diagnosis of constrictive pericarditis, although increased pericardial thickness is not present in all patients.

There are a number of pathological conditions that can be associated with equalization of ventricular diastolic pressures (Table 5)

Cardiac tamponade will have **elevated right-sided diastolic** pressures and low forward output resulting. As opposed to patients with constrictive pericarditis, **early diastolic rapid filling** will be blunted in patients with tamponade. Constrictive pericarditis is characterized by finding of early rapid filling and elevation with end equalization of diastolic pressures in all cardiac chambers (Table 5).

a) **Low pressure cardiac tamponade**: Any cause of severe depletion of intravascular volume (hemorrhage, diuresis or post dialysis) sometimes may have low pressure cardiac tamponade in which the intracardiac and pericardial diastolic pressures are only 6 to 12 mmHg. Diagnostic pulsus paradoxus may not be appreciated, but the hemodynamic significance of these effusions can be demonstrated on echocardiography by right heart chamber collapse and respiratory variations in transvalvular flows.

   A fluid challenge with a rapid infusion of one liter of isotonic saline in the catheterization laboratory will usually elicit typical cardiac tamponade hemodynamics. Echocardiographic abnormalities (e.g., size of the pericardial effusion, right sided chamber collapse, and exaggerated respiratory changes in mitral and tricuspid valve flow) are usually similar in frequency and magnitude to patients with classic cardiac tamponade. The spectrum of etiologies was similar to patients with classic cardiac tamponade.

   Clinical findings commonly associated with cardiac tamponade (eg, elevated heart rate, jugular venous distention, and pulsus paradoxus) were significantly less common in low pressure cardiac tamponade than in classic cardiac tamponade.

b) **Regional cardiac tamponade**: A loculated, eccentric effusion or localized hematoma can produce regional cardiac tamponade in which only selected chambers are compressed. As a result, the typical physical, hemodynamic, and echocardiographic signs of cardiac tamponade are often absent, including pulsus paradoxus, diastolic pressure equalization, and chamber compression in standard apical and parasternal views.

c) **Regional cardiac tamponade** is most often seen after pericardiotomy or myocardial infarction. Establishing the diagnosis is challenging and may require additional echocardiographic views (e.g., subcostal or transesophageal) and other advanced imaging techniques (e.g., computed tomography).

Acute Pulmonary Embolism

Patients with both a pericardial effusion and a pulmonary embolism are a clinical challenge. If they developed shock, the question becomes is this due to tamponade or a massive pulmonary embolism.

On physical exam, both groups of patients will have sinus tachycardia, hypotension, and an elevated JVP. Clinical finding to indicate tamponade in such patients may include muffled heart sounds, pericardial friction rub, and pulsus paradoxus. Note that a pulsus paradoxus can also be seen massive pulmonary embolism.

To differentiate between the two, bed side investigations in the form of ECG and bedside echocardiogram may be of help.

In patients with pulmonary embolism, ECG findings include:

- Sinus tachycardia
- Atrial arrhythmias
- S1Q3T3-rare but specific ECG pattern
- RBBB
- Right axis deviation
- Non-specific ST/T wave changes
- Precordial T-wave inversion (Right heart strain pattern)

Visualization with an echocardiogram would aid in putting this dilemma to rest. Findings on echocardiogram in massive pulmonary embolism include:

- Increased RV size
- Decreased RV function
- Tricuspid regurgitation

Right Ventricular Infarction

This condition may resemble cardiac tamponade with hypotension, elevated JVP, an absent Y descent in jugular venous pulse, occasionally pulsus paradoxus, and equalization of diastolic pressures may be present.

However, **Kussmaul's sign** and a third heart sound are usually present in right ventricular infarction distinguishing it from cardiac tamponade. Evaluation with an ECG and echocardiography will help confirm the diagnosis.

Cardiomyopathy with Congestive Heart Failure or with Cardiogenic Shock

This is one of the most common differential diagnoses of cardiac tamponade. Low blood pressure, tachycardia and elevated jugular venous pressure are common findings which mimic tamponade.

If chest x ray and ECG does not help to differentiate then urgent echocardiogram is warranted to make diagnosis of cardiac tamponade.

Investigation

CLINICAL PEARL 8 **EKG Findings in Tamponade:**
• Electrical alternans (seen in 20%) • Low Voltage (seen in 42%) • ± Signs of pericarditis • **Sinus tachycardia (most common)** • Pericarditis findings: ST elevation, PR depression

Electrocardiography (ECG)

None of the ECG findings in cardiac tamponade are pathognomic.

Sinus tachycardia is the major finding in ECG.Low QRS voltage (defined as maximum QRS amplitude <0.5 mV in the limb leads) was found in 61% of patients with cardiac tamponade.

Electrical alternans is recognized by alternating amplitude of the QRS complexes in any or all leads (Figure 7). Every other QRS complex has reduced amplitude alternating with increased amplitude. Most often it is observed in the precordial leads where the QRS amplitude is greater.

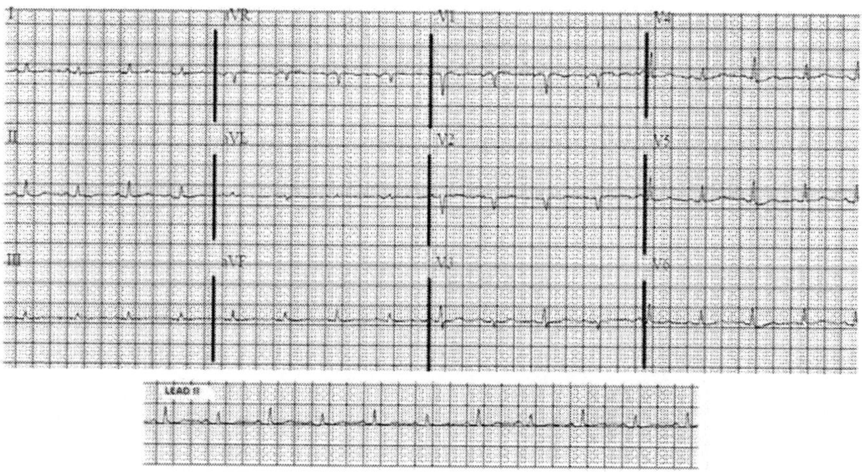

Figure 7. EKG showing low voltage wave and electrical alternans nicely demonstrated in lead II in zoom mode.

The *most frequent cause of electrical alternans is a pericardial effusion*; it is thought that the alternating amplitude is the result of a pendulum motion of the heart as it "swings" from beat to beat within the fluid contained in the pericardial sac; there is a change in electrical axis as the heart swings.

Electrical alternans may also be seen when there is severe cardiomegaly and left ventricular dysfunction and it may occur with aortic regurgitation.

Chest x-ray

Chest radiographs may show cardiomegaly with or without an epicardial fat pad sign suggesting a pericardial effusion (water bottle sign, Figure 8)).

The lungs are typically clear. However, chest radiographs may not be useful early in the course of the process, since at least 200 mL of pericardial fluid must accumulate before visible enlargement of the cardiac silhouette occurs.

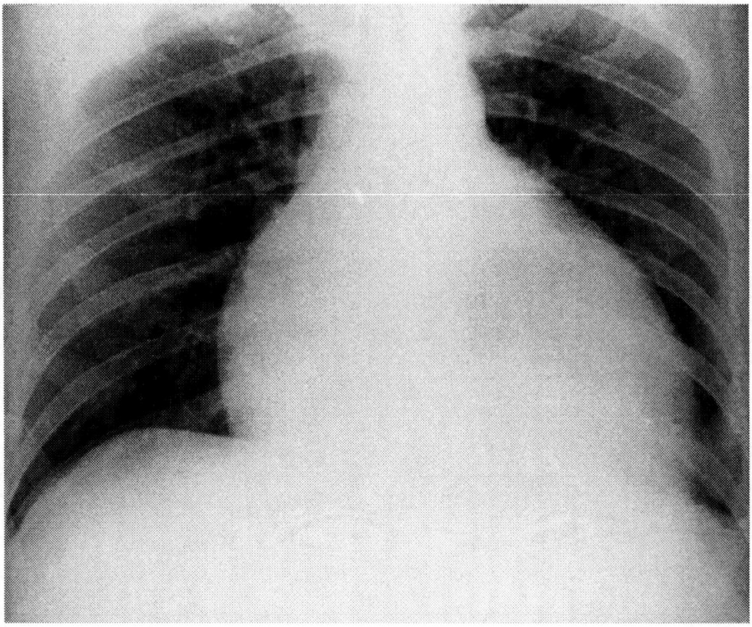

Figure 8. Chest x ray PA (posterior-anterior) view in patient with cardiac tamponade showing enlarged cardiac shadow (water bottle sign).

Acute cardiac tamponade can occur with a normal-size heart on chest radiographs especially after blunt chest trauma.

Paradoxically, patients with tamponade due to pneumopericardium or tension pneumopericardium, a substantial decrease in the size of the cardiac silhouette may be observed on radiographs, the small heart sign.

Transthoracic Echocardiography (TTE)

Transthoracic Echocardiography is the **most effective investigation** for the diagnosis of pericardial effusion, because it is sensitive, specific, noninvasive, and easily made available at the bedside.

Right atrial and right ventricular collapse are the most commonly used clues for tamponade at echocardiography; however, neither of them is 100% sensitive or specific for tamponade (Figure 9 & 10).

It also shows the size of effusion. Echocardiography can be used to visualize ventricular and atrial compression abnormalities as blood cycles through the heart. The following may be observed with 2-dimensional (2-D) echocardiography:

CLINICAL PEARL 9
Echocardiography is the diagnostic method of choice in suspected cardiac tamponade and should be carried out urgently.

- An echo-free space posterior and anterior to the left ventricle and behind the left atrium
- Early diastolic collapse of the right ventricular free wall
- Late diastolic compression/collapse of the right atrium
- Swinging of the heart in its sac
- Left Ventricular pseudohypertrophy
- Inferior vena cava plethora with minimal or no collapse with inspiration, may not be seen in low-pressure tamponade
- A greater than 40% relative inspiratory augmentation of right-side flow
- A greater than 25% relative decrease in inspiratory flow across the mitral valve

Echocardiography can also provide information on the significance of the pericardial effusion/tamponade. In the presence of cardiac tamponade, there is diastolic collapse of the free walls of the right atrium and/or right ventricle. This is due to compression of these relatively low-pressure structures by the higher-pressure pericardial effusion. As mentioned earlier, the thinner more compliant right-sided chambers are usually the first to be compressed in the setting of cardiac tamponade. *The collapse is exaggerated during expiration when right heart filling is reduced. Right a trial collapse is more sensitive for tamponade, but right ventricular collapse lasting more than one third of diastole is a more specific finding for cardiac tamponade.*

Of note, right ventricular collapse may also be present with large pleural effusions in the absence of pericardial effusion or cardiac tamponade. Persistence of right atrial inversion in ventricular systole is usually an early sign of cardiac tamponade, followed by diastolic compression of the right ventricular outflow tract. (Table 6)

Table 6. Major Echocardiographic Signs of Cardiac Tamponade

Signs	Sensitivity	Specificity
1. Large pericardial effusion with swinging heart	n.a.	n.a.
2. Diastolic collapse of right atrium (RA)	50–100%	33–100%
3. Duration of RA inversion by the RA inversion time index(duration of inversion/ cardiac cycle length); for values >0.34	>90%	100%
4. Diastolic collapse of right ventricle (RV)	48–100%	72–100%
5. Variations in E velocities during respiration across the mitral valve, tricuspid valve, and pulmonary outflow that are greater than 25, 50, and 30%.	n.a.	n.a.
6. Inferior vena cava (IVC) plethora (dilatation >20 mm and <50% reduction in the diameter of IVC with respiratory phases)	97%	40

European Heart Journal (2013) 34, 1186–1197 doi:10.1093/eurheartj/ehs372.

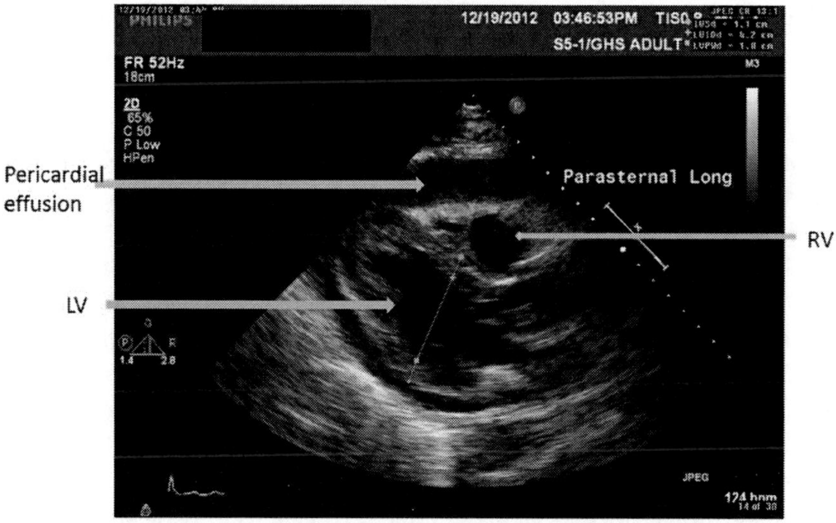

Transthoracic Echocardiogram done in a patient presented with progressive dyspnea: parasternal long axis showing large pericardial effusion
LV: left ventricle, RV: right ventricle

Figure 9.

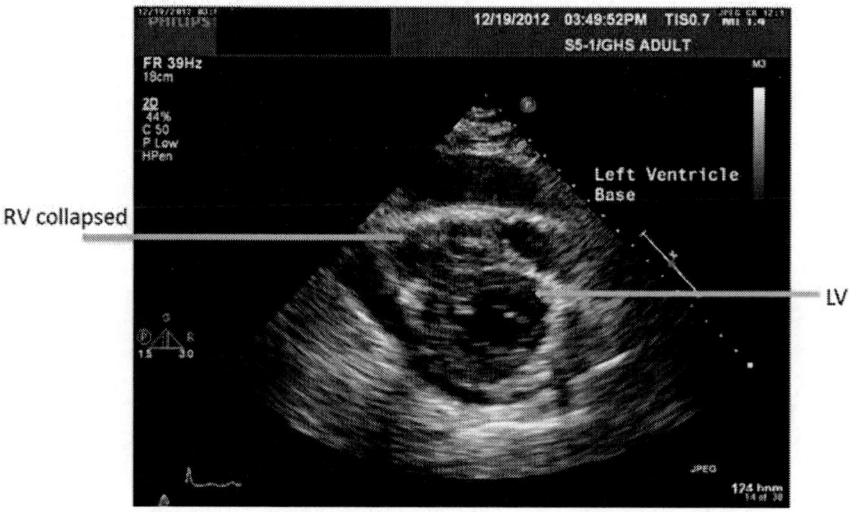

Figure 10.

Computed Tomography (CT) and Cardiovascular Magnetic Resonance (CMR)

CT and CMR can provide valuable aid in the search for *the cause of* pericardial effusions because they provide a larger field of view, allowing detection of loculated pericardial effusion, pericardial thickening and masses, as well as associated chest abnormalities.

CMR may also provide a combined morphological and functional evaluation. For both CT and CMR, the pericardium is ideal for imaging studies, because of a high natural contrast between pericardial layers separated by pericardial fluid, and contiguous fat tissue in the mediastinal and subepicardial space.

Both CCT and CMR provide more detailed quantification and localization of the effusion than TTE, and they are especially useful to guide pericardiocentesis, since loculated or regional effusions or regions of calcified pericardium can be identified. When hemopericardium complicates aortic dissection, CCT and CMR can readily identify the two diagnoses, thereby preventing inappropriate and potentially catastrophic pericardiocentesis.

CLINICAL PEARL 10 **About CT/CMR**
Not a part of the routine evaluation of patients with suspected cardiac tamponade. **Only useful to rule out concomitant diseases involving the mediastinum and lungs in patients with large pericardial effusions (i.e. cancer or aortic dissection).**

Some of the reported CT findings in tamponade include (nonspecific findings):

- superior vena cava enlargement
    - diameter similar to or greater than that of the adjacent thoracic aorta
- inferior vena cava enlargement

    - diameter greater than twice that of the adjacent abdominal aorta
- hepatic and renal vein enlargement
- periportal edema
- reflux of contrast material
    - into the Inferior Vena Cava
    - into the azygos system
- compression of the coronary sinus
- angulation or bowing of the interventricular septum

Cardiac Catheterization

Although not typically performed as the initial diagnostic test, cardiac catheterization can reveal two major findings in patients with cardiac tamponade: equilibration of average intracardiac diastolic pressures (usually between 10 and 30 mmHg) and the inspiratory increase in right-sided pressures and reduction in left-sided pressures that are responsible for pulsus paradoxus. Cardiac catheterization should be considered when any discrepancy is suspected between the clinical and non-invasive imaging data, and particularly in patients with complex hemodynamic disorders.

Treatment

Prompt recognition of cardiac tamponade is critical because the underlying hemodynamic disorder can lead to death if not resolved by percutaneous or surgical drainage of the pericardium.

When a pericardial effusion is detected, the first step is to evaluate its size and hemodynamic importance, as well as the possible association with concomitant diseases. Large idiopathic chronic effusion (> 3 months) have a 30-35% risk of progression to cardiac tamponade. Also subacute (4 to 6 weeks) large effusions not responsive to conventional therapy and with echocardiographic signs of right chambers collapse may have an increased risk of progression according to some authors who recommend preventive drainage in such cases.

If cardiac tamponade is diagnosed at a local hospital or primary care facility with limited experience in pericardiocentesis or in the presence of any of any it's contraindications and the patient is clinically stable to allow pericardiocentesis be delayed, the patient should be promptly transferred to a specialized institution.

If the patient is clinically unstable, pericardiocentesis cannot be delayed, then emergency pericardiocentesis becomes a life-saving procedure and should be performed under echo guidance. Pericardial drainage may not be necessary when the effusion is large but there is no hemodynamic impairment. It may resolve spontaneously or under anti-inflammatory treatment. Such cases with minimal symptoms and stable hemodynamic parameters may be observed with serial physical examinations and echocardiograms.

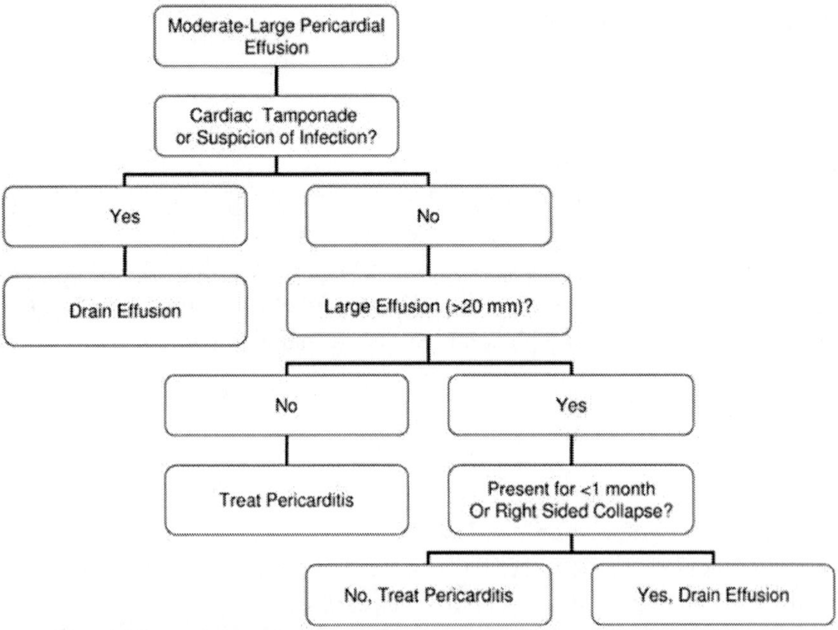

William C. Little, and Gregory L. Freeman Circulation. 2006;113:1622-1632

Figure 11.

An algorithm for managing patients with a moderate to large pericardial effusion has been proposed by Little et al in 2006 (Figure 11). However, a new comprehensive step-wise scoring system (European Society of Cardiology guidelines, 2014) has been proposed to provide additional support to clinicians about the selection of high risk patients that would need an immediate intervention and of those patients that should be transferred to specialized institutions (Figure 12). Per their recommendations, urgent surgical treatment of cardiac tamponade is needed, regardless of the score, in type A aortic dissection, ventricular free wall rupture after acute myocardial infarction, severe recent chest trauma, and iatrogenic hemopericardium when the bleeding cannot be controlled percutaneously.

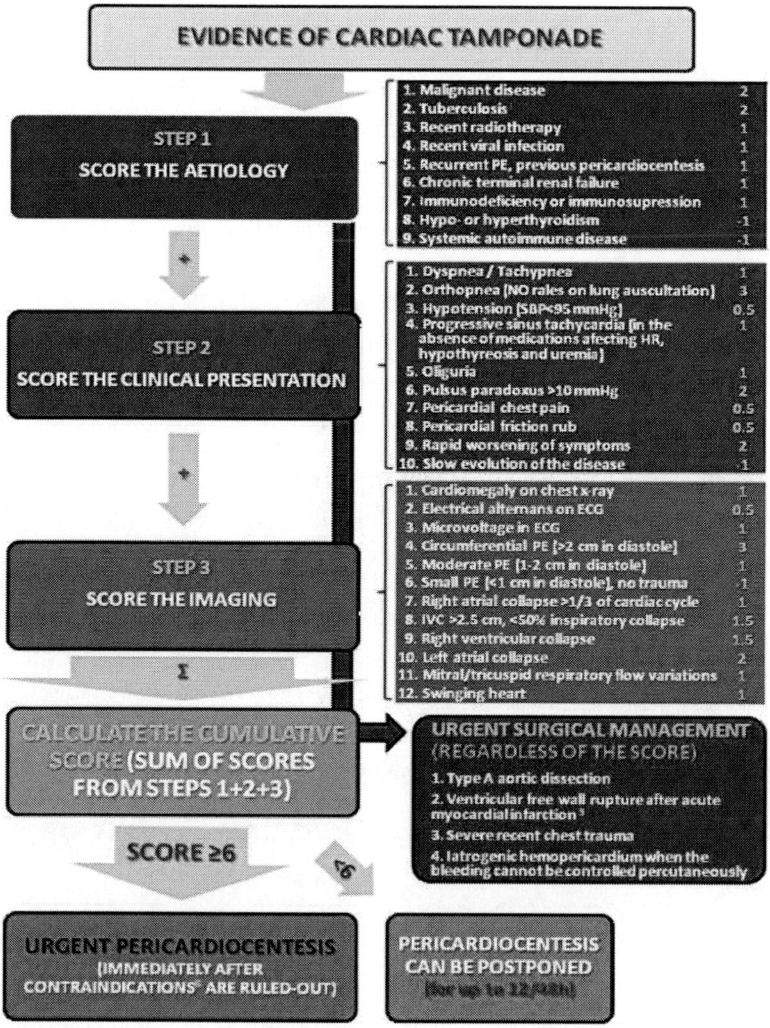

Figure 12. European Society of Cardiology scoring system (2014) of cardiac tamponade based on etiology, clinical presentation, and imaging. A score of 6 or greater requires urgent pericardiocentesis, while a score less than 6 can be postponed and patient may be transferred to specialized facility.

As most clinicians are not comfortable inserting a needle in to the pericardial sac, there may be a time delay until the procedure can be performed by a qualified expert. In that time, supportive measures and medical management of the underlying etiology should be initiated. Patients may require nonsteroidal anti-inflammatory drugs, colchicine, or steroids if idiopathic or viral pericarditis is suspected.

It is preferred for these patients to be monitored and taken care of in the intensive care unit, placed on bed rest with legs elevated to increase venous return, and receive oxygen. Furthermore, acidosis ought to be corrected, volume resuscitation with crystalloids or colloids such as blood or plasma should be administered in attempt to improve cardiac output, and vasopressor medications be given to improve perfusion pressure.

In significant tamponade, use of general anesthesia and positive-pressure ventilation may result in hypotension or cardiac arrest. This is attributable to anesthesia induced peripheral vasodilation, sympatholysis, changes in heart rate, and decreased venous return from increased intrathoracic pressure associated with mechanical ventilation.

Pericardiocentesis under local anesthesia is the preferred management in hypotensive patients with cardiac tamponade. Once fluid is removed and hemodynamic status has stabilized, sedation and mechanical ventilation can be instituted to permit surgical exploration for a more definitive treatment.

Pericardiocentesis I.E. Percutaneous Drainage versus Surgical Approach to Drain the Fluid

Removal of pericardial fluid is the definitive therapy for tamponade and can be done using the following approaches in different clinical scenarios:

- Emergency subxiphoid percutaneous drainage or “blind” technique
- Echocardiographically guided pericardiocentesis
- Pericardiotomy (either surgical or percutaneous balloon pericardiostomy)

Pericardial fluid removal can be accomplished by catheter or needle pericardiocentesis, open surgical drainage with or without pericardiectomy (pericardial "window"), or video-assisted thoracoscopicpericardiectomy.

Ultrasound Guided Pericardiocentesis

The procedure of pericardiocentesis underwent a reform with the introduction of the ultrasound or echocardiography-guided pericardiocentesis in the late 1970s. Most patients with tamponade will require early drainage of the pericardial effusion which is the definitive way to relieve the elevated intrapericardial pressure and improving hemodynamic status.

Table 7. Three Approaches of Pericardiocentesis

Technique	Description	Pros	Cons
Parasternal	• Needle inserted close to the sternum • 5th intercostal space	• Pericardium exposed at site of cardiac notch of left lung • Commonly used with echocardiogram guidance	• Higher risk of Pneumothorax • Internal thoracic vessels at risk of injury as close to sternal margin
Subxiphoid	• Needle inserted into angle between xiphisternum and left costal margin, directed towards left shoulder	• Safest approach in emergent situation when ultrasound not available • Less risk of pleural injury	• Highest rate of morbidity and mortality • Diaphragm and phrenic nerve irritation • Higher risk of liver injury • Risk of Colon/Stomach Perforation
Apical	• Needle placed 1cm outside apex beat in intercostal space, directed towards right shoulder	• Thick left ventricular wall • Pericardium is superficial • Area over cardiac apex is bare, pleura is usually absent • Patient in left lateral position allows accumulation of fluid around apex	• Higher risk of ventricular fibrillation • Not indicated in emergency situations

Transthoracicechocardiography needs to be performed urgently for the assessment of pericardial effusion because these patients might require prompt drainage and placement of an indwelling pericardial catheter. **Catheter pericardiocentesis with the help of echocardiography** is treatment of choice in most patients, which is also recommended in 2004 European Society of Cardiology guidelines on pericardial disease.

Echo-guided pericardiocentesis is the minimal invasive procedure and has become the best option to manage cardiac tamponade because of lower complication and mortality rates especially in idiopathiccases and in patients with hemodynamic instability. However, loculation with fibrin accumulation may occur resulting in a pericardial empyema, making percutaneous drainage incomplete and ineffective. In such cases, a pericardial window or extensive pericardiectomy usually through subxiphoid pericardiotomy is essential to achieve adequate drainage.

There are **three commonly described** techniques for pericardiocentesis; the left parasternal, subxyphoid and apical approach, each with its own pros and cons, and used depending on how urgent the situation (Table 7).

1. Left Parasternal Approach

In a hemodynamically stable patient, the left parasternal approach (Figure 13), with ultrasound guidance, provides the most controlled approach to pericardiocentesis, and avoids structures such as the diaphragm and phrenic nerve. It provides a more direct route to the largest echo free space and better safety than other approaches.

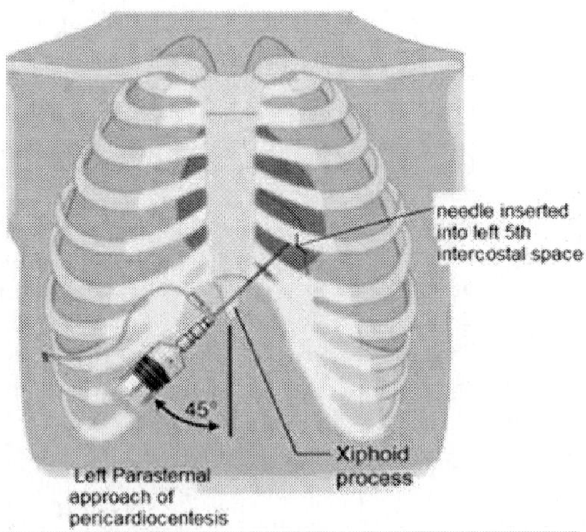

Figure 13. Parasternal Approach.

Using this approach, the puncture needle is inserted close to the sternum, usually in the left 4th to 6th intercostal space where the largest fluid collection is present closest to the skin.

2. Subxyphoid Approach

The needle in this approach is inserted at an angle between the xiphisternum and left costal margin, towards the left shoulder at a 15 to 30 degree angle to the skin Figure 14. *It is exclusively used as blind technique.* This approach has been highly discouraged and may be considered only when echocardiography is not available, or in emergent situations.

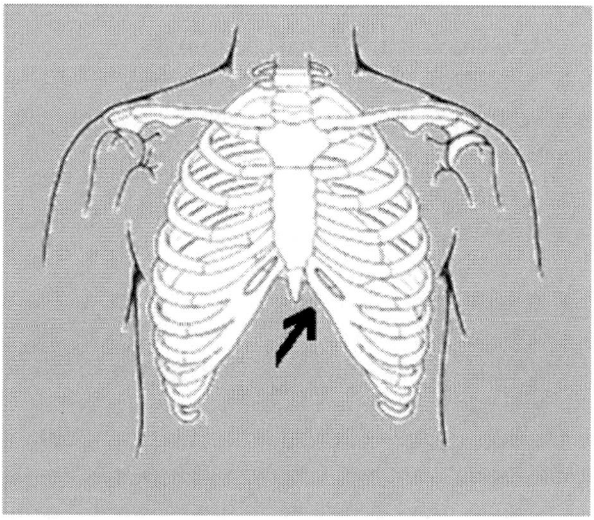

Figure 14. SubxyphoidApproach (*arrow pointing*).

This route is extrapleural and avoids the coronary, pericardial, and internal mammary arteries. Injuries to the pleura, liver, or stomach, irritation to the diaphragm and phrenic nerve resulting in bradycardia and shock, and higher procedure-related mortality have been reported with this approach than with others though the risk of pleura injury is less than other parasternal approach.

3. Left Apical Approach

The needle is inserted into the intercostal space outside of the left nipple, where the left ventricular apical beat is felt, and is directed towards the right shoulder. To allow fluid to accumulate around the apex of the heart, the patient should be positioned in the left posterior oblique position. This location is close to the lingual of the lung and left pleural space, but there lies a bare area over the cardiac apex where the pleura are usually absent.

The pericardial sac is superficial here with a relatively large transverse diameter, and therefore needle insertion has minimal risk to injure the pleura, myocardium, liver or lung. However during this approach, the apex can easily be pierced, and evoke ventricular fibrillation; thus, it is not indicated in emergent situations and must be performed under the guidance of echocardiography.

The choice of direction of approach must be decided by an experienced clinician, after considering if there is a safe enough margin of echo free space, the patient's position, and clinical situation.

During pericardiocentesis, clinicians must be attentive to the important anatomic structures in the way of the puncture needle approach, including the internal thoracic arteries (located 0.5 to 2 cm lateral to the sternal edge), intercostal vessels (inferior border of the rib) and nerves, phrenic nerve in the diaphragm, pleura, lung parenchyma, and free wall of the right or left ventricle.

EKG Changes during Pericardiocentesis

There may be ECG changes that may help the clinician know when the needle touches the myocardium. ST segment elevation or PR segment elevation may be seen if there is contact between the needle and an intact pericardium immediately overlying the heart with no fluid in the pericardial sac. However, if bloody fluid is obtained from the needle in the absence of these ECG changes, it signifies that fluid has been obtained from the pericardial space and not from the chambers of the heart. If the ECG reveals marked ST segment elevation or ventricular ectopic beats it signifies the needle touching the ventricle.

Atrial dysrrhythmias, change of P-wave morphology, elevation of the PR segment, atrial arrhythmias or atrioventricular dissociation may all be seen if there is contact with the atrium.

Complications

A number of complications may occur while guiding a needle into the pericardial space that the clinician should be aware of.

As stated earlier, it is of great benefit to visualize and quantify the amount of fluid between the myocardium and the pericardium. Needle insertion at the site of most fluid between the two will have the least risk of complication. One of the most common complications of pericardiocentesis occurs due to the needle touching or penetrating the myocardium.

The majority of perforations occur at the site of the right ventricle. Though most right ventricular perforations are without adverse effect, some have led to fatalities. The right ventricle is more susceptible to laceration as it is thinner than the left ventricle. With puncture of the ventricle there is always possibility of developing hemopericardium, another life threatening condition.

Other complications of pericardiocentesis worth noting include cardiac arrhythmias, pneumothorax, hemothorax, puncture of the right atrium, vascular injury to the coronary, intercostal, internal mammary, or intra-abdominal vessel, liver injury, stomach or colon perforation, and infection.

Open Surgical Approach

It might be preferred for traumatic cases, purulent pericarditis, or with recurrent malignant pericardial effusions. If the pericardial effusion cannot be reached by a needle or a catheter, **surgical drainage** is required, usually through a subcostal incision. **Open surgical drainage** may be done with or without pericardiectomy (pericardial "window"), or video-assisted thoracoscopic pericardiectomy with a beside catheter pericardiocentesis.

Aortic dissection and post-infarction rupture of the free wall are indications for urgent surgical drainage that should not be delayed in anyway by pericardiocentesis. If the surgical management of the aortic dissection is not promptly available or the patient is too unstable to survive the transfer to surgery, pericardiocentesis and controlled pericardial drainage of very small amounts of the hemopericardium can be attempted to temporarily stabilize the patient.

Open surgical drainage has the additional benefit of resecting a portion of the pericardium for histological examination, breaking up loculations, evacuation of hematoma, and placing a large drainage tube, which is especially important in purulent pericarditis.

The disadvantages of the open surgical procedures remain a) general anesthesia (risk of sudden hypotension in patients with large effusions/cardiac tamponade), b) a need to perform a 6- to 8-cm vertical incision in the upper abdomen as well as to resect the xiphoid process in some cases.

Evaluation of the Pericardial Fluid

The appropriate diagnostic tests to consider for the pericardial fluid vary according to the suspected etiology of the effusion. A more detailed discussion of pericardial fluid analysis is presented in table 8.

Table 8. Routine analyses of Pericardial fluid

Analysis	Test	Etiology or feature
General chemistry[a]	• Specific gravity. >1015 • Protein level >3 g/dL, Protein fluid/ serum ratio >0.5 • LDH >200 mg/dL, LDH Fluid/serum ratio >0.6 • Glucose • Blood cell count	**Exudate**
Cytology	Cytology (higher volumes of fluid, centrifugation, and rapid analysis improve diagnostic yield)	Cancer
Biomarkers	Tumour markers (i.e. CEA >5 ng/mL or CYFRA 21-1 >100 ng/mL) Adenosine deaminase >40 U/ L, IFN-gamma	Cancer TBC
Polymerase chain reaction (PCR)	PCR for specific infectious agents (i.e. TBC)	TBC
Microbiology	Acid-fast bacilli staining, mycobacterium cultures, aerobic, and anaerobic cultures	TBC Other bacteria

LDH, lactate dehydrogenase; TBC, tuberculosis.

a: These chemical features have been especially validated for pleural fluid and not pericardial fluid, although generally used also for pericardial effusion.

European Heart Journal (2013) 34, 1186–1197 doi:10.1093/eurheartj/ehs372

While pericardial fluid drainage in the setting of cardiac tamponade is done primarily for its therapeutic benefit, the procedure may also be diagnostic, particularly in patients with an uncertain etiology for the effusion. Obviously, the diagnostic work-up needs to be guided by the epidemiology and the clinical presentation to avoid performing extensive and unnecessary tests.

Non-idiopathic and non-viral etiologies (especially bacterial and neoplastic) are associated with an increased risk of cardiac tamponade and large effusion, and pericardiocentesis is mandatory when cardiac tamponade or such etiologies are suspected.

Cytology and tumour markers [carcinoembryonic antigen (CEA), alfa-feto protein, carbohydrate antigens CA 125, CA 72-4, CA 15-3, CA 19-9, etc.) should be performed in suspected malignant disease.

As already mentioned, developing countries have a high rate of pericardial effusions correlated to tuberculosis that should be ruled out in immigrants from endemic region of tuberculosis and HIV-infected patients.

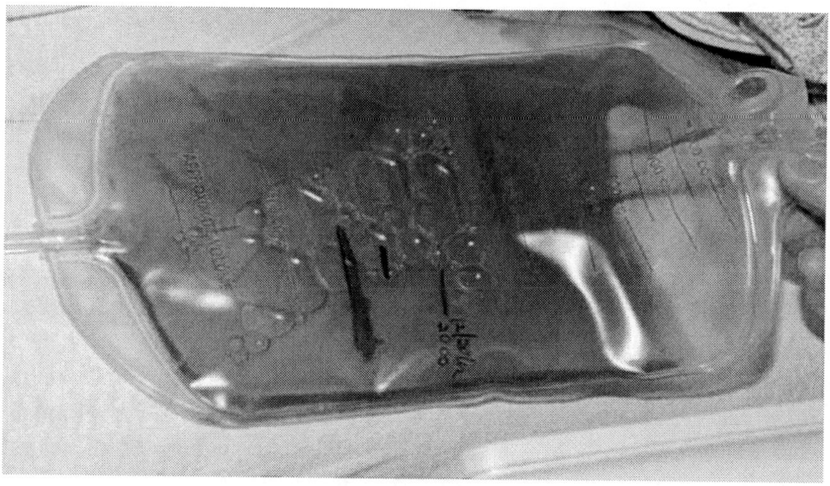

Figure 15. Green purulent fluid was retrieved after emergency large-volume pericardiocentesis done in 62 year old man who presented with features of cardiac tamponade. Symptoms started a week prior his arrival to the hospital. The culture grew polymicrobial organisms. However, primary source of infection was not identified.

In suspected tuberculosis acid-fast bacilli staining, mycobacterium culture or radiometric growth detection (e.g. BACTEC-460), adenosine deaminase (ADA), interferon (IFN)-gamma, pericardial lysozyme, and as well as PCR analyses for tuberculosis should be performed.

Differentiation of tuberculous and neoplastic effusion is virtually absolute with low levels of ADA and high levels of CEA. In addition, high ADA levels may predict the evolution towards pericardial constriction. In suspected bacterial infections, at least three cultures of pericardial fluid for aerobes and anaerobes as well as the blood cultures are mandatory.

Analysis of pericardial effusion can establish the diagnosis of infectious and neoplastic pericardial effusions. Sometime gross appearance of pericardial fluid helps to differentiate infectious versus neoplastic etiology Figure 15. Primary purulent pericardial tamponade revealing green pericardial fluid has been discussed in literature.

PCR analyses for cardiotropic viruses have been suggested, but are rarely used in clinical practice. Analyses of the pericardial fluid specific gravity (1015), protein level (3.0 g/dL), fluid/serum ratio (0.5), LDH (200 mg/dL), serum/fluid (0.6), and glucose can separate exudates from transudates, but are not directly diagnostic. Nevertheless, purulent effusions with positive cultures have significantly lower fluid glucose levels than non-infectious effusions. White cell count is highest in inflammatory and infectious diseases, and lowest in myxedema.

Pericardial Window or Pericardiectomy via Balloon or Surgical Approach

Surgical drainage has the advantages of permitting diagnostic pericardial biopsies to be taken and pericardiectomy to be performed, if needed. Direct surgical visualization may also be preferable if fluid has re-accumulated after catheter drainage, the effusion is loculated, there is a special need for biopsy material, or the patient has a coagulopathy. However, surgical drainage requires general anesthesia, which may worsen hemodynamic compromise if needle drainage is not performed first to reduce the severity of the cardiac tamponade.

If the pericardial effusion cannot be reached by a needle or a catheter, surgical drainage is required, usually through a subcostal incision. Furthermore, surgical drainage is desirable in patients with purulent pericardial fluid, intrapericardial bleeding, and in those with clotted hemopericardium or thoracic conditions that make pericardiocentesis difficult or ineffective.

Pericardial Biopsy

Pericardial biopsy is generally reserved for cases with recurrent cardiac tamponade or persistence without a defined etiology, especially when a bacterial or neoplastic etiology is suspected and cannot be assessed by other conventional and less invasive means.

Technical advances in instrumentation, introduction of pericardioscopy and contemporary pathology, virology, and molecular biology techniques have improved the diagnostic value of epicardial/pericardial biopsy.

Pericardioscopy performed through air instead of fluid, made it possible to inspect large areas of pericardial surface, select the biopsy site, and take numerous samples. Targeted pericardial/epicardial biopsy during pericardioscopy was particularly useful in the diagnosis of neoplastic pericarditis.

No major complications were reported with the use of flexible pericardioscopies. Such techniques and approaches are warranted in skilled tertiary referral centers for selected cases, when a specific diagnosis, that may require a targeted therapy (i.e. neoplastic pericardial effusion), is suspected and cannot be diagnosed by traditional diagnostic means.

Intrapericardial Fibrinolysis

As there is no consensus exists on the optimal management of purulent tamponade, few authors propose intrapericardial fibrinolysis, a less invasive procedure as an alternative to surgery.

It is believed that frequent irrigation of the pericardial cavity with urokinase or streptokinase using large catheters might liquefy the purulent exudate, but there is a lack of good quality of evidence as a treatment for purulent pericarditis and for prevention of its recurrence and development of constrictive pericarditis.

Meanwhile, in retrospective studies, as compared to simple drainage, systematic pericardiectomy can prevent the occurrence of constrictive pericarditis with a better clinical outcome. It has to be emphasized here that the cornerstone of purulent pericarditis management includes the complete eradication of the primary focus of infection.

Special Considerations for the Management of Neoplastic Pericardial Effusions

After the appropriate drainage procedure, it is essential that treating physicians make a further treatment plan in the context of the cancer stage, the patient's prognosis, the success rates and risks of the various modalities, and local availability and expertise.

Since cardiac tamponade with underlying malignancy easily recur, various approaches have been proposed to prevent the long term recurrences. In such cases, different approaches such as extended drainage, pericardial window (either surgical or percutaneous balloon pericardiostomy), sclerosing local therapy, local and/or systemic chemotherapy or radiation therapy have been discussed in the literature.

The ultimate outcomes of various therapeutic approaches depend on different tumor types. Lymphomas and leukemias can be treated with systemic chemotherapy; for solid tumors, percutaneous drainage and the use of systemic and/or local sclerosing and antineoplastic therapy seems to offer the best chance of success.

The agents that can work as both sclerosing and antineoplastic activity such as bleomycin or thiotepa are quite effective in breast cancer, at least when associated with systemic chemotherapy. Local chemotherapy with platinum, mitoxantrone and other agents can be used for good local control of the disease and improve survival. The rationale of use of antineoplastic agents is to cure the local metastases, rather than simply prevent effusion by sclerosis.

Meanwhile, intrapericardial treatment tailored to the type of cancer indicates that cisplatin is more effective in secondary lung cancer, whereas thiotepa seems to be effective in breast cancer. Surgical or percutaneous pericardiostomy and radiation therapy may be useful in recurring effusions or cases not responding to other treatments.

Relative Contraindications to Pericardial Fluid Drainage

While pericardiocentesis can be safely performed in most patients, there are situations in which the procedure may need to be postponed.

Severe pulmonary hypertension – Caution must be taken if pericardiocentesis is performed in patients with severe pulmonary hypertension. In the setting of severe pulmonary hypertension, the pericardial effusion may be preventing significant dilatation of the right ventricle, which may be crucial to supporting the right ventricle. Drainage of the pericardial fluid may lead to loss of this support of the right ventricle, causing worsening of right ventricular function and more severe tricuspid regurgitation.

Bleeding diathesis/coagulopathy – The relative risks and benefits of pericardiocentesis should also be closely considered if a bleeding diathesis or coagulopathy is present such as INR >1.5, thrombocytopaenia (especially when platelet count <50,000/mm3). Although the risk of complications is low, bleeding risk is higher in the setting of coagulopathy. In addition, the subcostal approach should be avoided in the setting of a coagulopathy as bleeding from liver injury can be life threatening.

In most cases, however, the potential benefits for a patient with significant hemodynamic compromise related to cardiac tamponade will outweigh the risks associated with the procedure.

Prognosis and Complications

The prognosis of pericardial tamponade is essentially related to the etiology, and thus it is important to identify specific etiology that requires targeted therapies. The overall mortality risk depends on the speed of diagnosis, the treatment provided, and the underlying cause of the tamponade. If untreated, the condition is rapidly and universally fatal.

In a study of patients with cardiac tamponade, Cornily et al., reported a 1-year mortality rate of 76.5% in patients whose tamponade was caused by malignant disease, compared with 13.3% in patients with no malignant disease. The investigators also noted a median survival of 150 days in patients with malignant disease.

Malignant pericardial effusions are associated with poor prognosis. Hence, it is important for clinicians to focus on reducing symptoms and improving the quality of life as primary goals of treatment in patients presenting with malignant pericardial effusions. Management of these patients requires multidisciplinary approaches with cooperation between cardiologists, cardiac surgeons, oncologists, radiotherapists and palliative care physicians.

The size of the effusion is also correlates to the prognosis, because moderate to large effusions are more common for specific etiologies such as bacterial, neoplastic or related to a systemic inflammatory disease. Bacterial etiologies as well as post-radiation pericardial diseases, pericardial injury syndromes have an increased risk of developing complications either early or intermediate (cardiac tamponade, recurrences) or late (constrictive pericarditis). Idiopathic pericardial tamponade has an overall good prognosis with a very low risk of complications if the tamopanade is managed emergently.

Acknowledgment

We would like to thank Dr. Eman Alsharif, Dr. Samir Amr (Pathology Consultant, KSA), Sami Amr PHD (Harvard Lab director, USA), Dr. Ziad Issa (Cardiology Consultant, USA), Hitekshya Nepal MD (Resident, SIU-school of medicine, USA) for their time and hard work to accomplish this project.

Conflict of interest: *None*

References

[1] Gumrukcuoglu HA, Odabasi D, Akdag S, Ekim H. Management of Cardiac Tamponade: A Comparative Study between Echo-Guided Pericardiocentesis and Surgery-A Report of 100 Patients. *Cardiol Res Pract* 2011; 2011:197838.

[2] Sagristà-Sauleda J, Angel J, Sambola A, et al. Low-pressure cardiac tamponade: clinical and hemodynamic profile. *Circulation* 2006; 114:945.

[3] Spodick DH. Acute cardiac tamponade. *N Engl J Med* 2003; 349:684.

[4] Yared K1, Baggish AL, Picard MH, Hoffmann U, Hung. Multimodality imaging of pericardial diseases. *JACC Cardiovasc Imaging*. 2010 Jun;3(6):650-60.

[5] Oliver Navarrete C, Marín Ortuño F, Pineda Rocamora J, Luján Martínez J, García Fernández A, et al. .Should we Try to Determine the Specific Cause of Cardiac Tamponade? *Rev Esp Cardiol.* 2002 May;55(5):493-8.

[6] Cornily JC, Pennec PY, Castellant P, Bezon E, Le Gal G, Gilard M, et al. Cardiac tamponade in medical patients: a 10-year follow-up survey. *Cardiology*. 2008;111(3):197-201.

[7] Permanyer-Miralda G, Sagristá-Sauleda J, Soler-Soler J: Primary acute pericardial disease: a prospective series of 231 consecutive patients. *Am J Cardiol* 1985; 56:623-630.

[8] Campbell P, Leopold JA, Selwyn AP, Sisto D. Equalization of right- and left-sided intracardiac pressures: is it constriction? *Circulation: Heart Failure*. 2011; 4: 374-377

[9] Lorell, BH, Grossman, W. Profiles in constrictive pericarditis, restrictive cardiomyopathy, and cardiac tamponade. in: W Grossman (Ed.) *Cardiac catheterization and angiography*. Lea & Febiger, Philadelphia; 1986:427–445.

[10] Bhattarai M, Yost G, Good CW, White CF, Nepal H. Primary Purulent Pericarditis with Cardiac Tamponade due to Oropharyngeal Polymicrobial Infection: A Case Report and Literature Review. *Korean J Thorac Cardiovasc Surg*. 2014 Apr;47(2):155-9.

[11] Imazio M, Adler Y. Management of pericardial effusion. *Eur Heart J*. 2013 Apr;34(16):1186-97.

[12] Little WC, Freeman GL. Pericardial disease. *Circulation*. 2006 Mar 28;113(12):1622-32.

[13] Mookadam, F., Jiamsripong, P., Oh, J. K., & Khandheria, B. K. (2009). *Spectrum of pericardial disease: part I*, 1149-1157.

[14] Roy, C. L., Minor, M. A., Brookhart, M. A., & Choudhry, N. K. (2007). Does this patient with a pericardial effusion have cardiac tamponade?. *JAMA*, 297(16), 1810-1818.

[15] Asher, C. R., & Klein, A. L. (2002). Diastolic heart failure: restrictive cardiomyopathy, constrictive pericarditis, and cardiac tamponade: clinical and echocardiographic evaluation. *Cardiology in review*, 10(4), 218-229.

[16] Dunne, J. V., Chou, J. P., Viswanathan, M., Wilcox, P., & Huang, S. H. (2011). Cardiac tamponade and large pericardial effusions in systemic sclerosis. *Clinical rheumatology*, 30(3), 433-438.

[17] Swami, A., & Spodick, D. H. (2003). Pulsus paradoxus in cardiac tamponade: a pathophysiologic continuum. *Clinical cardiology*, 26(5), 215-217.

[18] Schiavone, W. A. (2013). Cardiac tamponade: 12 pearls in diagnosis and management. *Cleveland Clinic journal of medicine*, 80(2), 109-116.

[19] Aikat, S., & Ghaffari, S. (2000). A review of pericardial diseases: clinical, ECG and hemodynamic features and management. *Cleveland Clinic journal of medicine*, 67(12), 903-914.

[20] Schairer, J. R., Biswas, S., Keteyian, S. J., & Ananthasubramaniam, K. A systematic approach to evaluation of pericardial effusion and cardiac tamponade. *Cardiology in review*, 19(5), 233-238.

[21] Spodick, D. H. (1992). Macrophysiology, microphysiology, and anatomy of the pericardium: a synopsis. *American heart journal*, 124(4), 1046-1051.

[22] Hoit, B. D. Pericardial disease and pericardial tamponade. *Critical care medicine*, (2007), 35(8), S355-S364.

[23] Braunwald, E., Zipes, D. P., & Libby P, eds. *Heart disease: a textbook of cardiovascular medication,* 6(2), (pp. 1823-1876). Philadelphia, PA: W.B. Saunders.

[24] Reddy, P. S., Curtiss, E. I., & Uretsky, B. F. (1990). Spectrum of hemodynamic changes in cardiac tamponade. *The American journal of cardiology*, 66(20), 1487-1491.

[25] Maisch, B., Seferović, P. M., Ristić, A. D., Erbel, R., Rienmüller, R., Adler, et.al. Guidelines on the diagnosis and management of pericardial diseases executive summary The Task force on the diagnosis and management of pericardial diseases of the European society of cardiology. *European Heart Journal*, (2004). 25(7), 587-610.

[26] Le Winter M. M., Kabbani S. (2005). Pericardial diseases. In: Zipes, D. P., Libby, P., Bonow, R. O., & Braunwald, E, eds. *Braunwald's Heart Disease.* 7, (pp. 1757-1780). Philadelphia, PA: Elsevier Saunders.

[27] Miyazaki, T., Pride, H. P., & Zipes, D. P. (1990). Prostaglandins in the pericardial fluid modulate neural regulation of cardiac electrophysiological properties. *Circulation research*, 66(1), 163-175.

[28] Applegate, R. J., Johnston, W. E., Vinten-Johansen, J. A. K. O. B., Klopfenstein, H. S., & Little, W. C. (1992). Restraining effect of intact pericardium during acute volume loading. *American Journal of Physiology-Heart and Circulatory Physiology,* 262(6), H1725-H1733.

[29] Spodick, D. H. (1997). The Pericardium: A Comprehensive Textbook. (pp. 7-14). NY: Marcel Dekker.

[30] Perera, P., Lobo, V., Williams, S. R., & Gharahbaghian, L. (2014) Cardiac Echocardiography. *Critical Care Clinics*, 30(1), 47-92.

[31] Sorajja P. Invasive hemodynamics of constrictive pericarditis, restrictive cardiomyopathy, and cardiac tamponade. *Cardiol Clin.* 2011 May;29(2):191-9.

[32] Corey GR, Campbell PT, Van Trigt P, Kenney RT, O'Connor CM, Sheikh KH, Kisslo JA, Wall TC. Etiology of large pericardial effusions. *Am J Med.* 1993 Aug;95(2):209-13.

[33] BP & Pulsus Paradoxus, #17 BP & Pulsus Paradoxus, Date Accessed: March 19, 2015 http://stanfordmedicine25.stanford.edu/the25/bppp.html.
[34] Ristić AD, Imazio M, Adler Y, Anastasakis A, Badano LP. et al. Triage strategy for urgent management of cardiac tamponade: a position statement of the European Society of Cardiology Working Groupon Myocardial and Pericardial Diseases. *Eur Heart J.* 2014 Sep 7;35(34):2279-84.
[35] Jung HO. *Pericardial effusion and pericardiocentesis: role of echocardiography. Korean Circ J.* 2012 Nov;42(11):725-34
[36] Chatterjee K. Response to Campbell: Is This a Case of Constriction? Circulation: Heart Failure. 2011; 4: 374-377. doi: 10.1161/CIRCHEARTFAILURE.111.961276
[37] https://web.stanford.edu/group/ccm_echocardio/cgi-bin/mediawiki/index.php/Tamponade

In: Cardiac Tamponade
Editor: Cameron L. Pittman

ISBN: 978-1-63482-787-4

Chapter 2

Cardiac Tamponade: Etiology, Hemodynamics, and Management

Rina R. Shah, Simon K. Topalian and M. Rizwan Sardar*
Cooper University Hospital, Camden, NJ,
Department of Cardiology/3rd Floor Dorrance,
One Cooper Plaza Camden, NJ

The pericardium is composed of two layers – the visceral pericardium and fibrous parietal layer, and it contains a thin layer of fluid surrounding the heart. When larger amounts of fluid accumulate under pressure or when the pericardium is scarred and inelastic, one of three pericardial compressive syndromes may occur.

Cardiac tamponade may be characterized by chronicity of fluid buildup and variant of pressure. Hemodynamic response in cardiac tamponade depends on the pressure in the pericardial sac and the ability of the heart to compensate for elevated pressure, which is directly related to the amount of fluid and the pericardial pressure-volume relation. With cardiac tamponade, all of the

* Corresponding author: M. Rizwan Sardar, M Cooper University Hospital, Camden, NJ, Department of Cardiology/3rd Floor Dorrance, One Cooper Plaza Camden, NJ 08103, rizwansardar@hotmail.com.

cardiac chambers are compressed due to increased pericardial pressure. Ultimately, cardiac chamber diastolic compliance is compromised.

Constrictive pericarditis is the result of scarring and eventual inelasticity of the pericardial sac. This results in markedly restricted filling of the heart, causing an elevation and equilibration of filling pressures in all chambers of the heart along with systemic and pulmonary veins.

In both cardiac tamponade and constrictive pericarditis, cardiac filling is impeded. The normal pericardium is able to stretch to accommodate physiologic changes in cardiac volume. However, after reaching the reserve volume, the pericardium stiffens. There will be enhanced ventricular interaction or interdependence.

Effusive-constrictive pericarditis combines an underlying effusion or tamponade with an underlying constrictive physiology. The physical, hemodynamic, and echocardiographic findings are generally a mixture of those associated with tamponade and constrictive pericarditis.

Treatment modalities vary depending on the type of pericardial compressive syndrome diagnosed. While some patients may benefit from a pericardiocentesis, others may require a definitive surgical treatment such as pericardiectomy.

Normal Pericardial Anatomy

The normal pericardium is composed of two layers and is a rigid, avascular fibrous sac. The inner layer, known as the visceral pericardium, is comprised of a single layer of serous membrane and is continuous with the epicardial surface of the heart. The membrane is comprised of mesothelial cells, collagen and elastin fibers. The outer fibrous pericardial layer is a dense but thin fibrous structure with elastin fibrils and is apposed to the pleural surfaces. The pericardial space is defined as the space between the two layers and typically consists a small amount of serious fluid, generally between 5-10 mL, which may be detectable by echocardiography.

The pericardium is normally a rigid and noncompliant structure that predominantly acts to limit cardiac chamber distention with changes in volume, which contributes to ventricular stiffness in diastole. The cardiac chambers interact via the interventricular septum. Due to the noncompliant nature of the pericardium, when there is an accumulation of fluid in the pericardial space, there is a rapid rise in pericardial pressure. The amount of volume that can be accommodated by the pericardial space without increasing pericardial pressure is known as the pericardial reserve volume and is generally around 50-75 mL. Pericardial fluid is normally drained via the right lymphatic and thoracic ducts.

When the fluid accumulates gradually, the pericardium stretches and remodels, allowing a greater pericardial reserve volume. Once the pericardial reserve volume is reached, any additional fluid accumulation will result in rapid pressure increases in the pericardial space. This is the basis of the *last-drop effect*, in which a small amount of fluid can cause hemodynamic compromise or a small amount of fluid removal can lead to rapid improvement. [1, 2]

Normal Pericardial Physiology

The interactions between the pericardium, pericardial space, cardiac cambers, and thoracic cavity during the cardiac and respiratory cycles are quite complex. The pericardial space is found within the thoracic cavity, which has a normal pressure ranging from -6 to 0 mm Hg.[1] The true filling pressure is the myocardial transmural pressure, which is defined as the intracardiac pressure minus the pericardial pressure. [2] Pericardial compliance and the total intrapericardial volume govern pericardial pressure. [3]

The cardiac chambers are located within the pericardial space, whereas the pulmonary veins exist outside the pericardial space but within the thoracic cavity. The superior vena cava and inferior vena cava also exist outside the pericardial space, but are partially within the thoracic cavity. Thus, the systemic venous circulation is independent of changes in the intrathoracic pressures.

Normally, during inspiration, the intrathoracic pressure decreases, causing a pressure drop in the right heart, thereby increasing right heart filling. During inspiration, the pressure within the pulmonary veins also falls. With the pressure decreasing throughout the left atrium, left ventricle, and pulmonary veins during inspiration, there is no major change in left ventricular (LV) filling pattern. Therefore, during inspiration, the septum bows from right to left due to increased right ventricular (RV) filling and no change in LV filling. This results in impaired left-sided cardiac output, which causes a small, inspiratory drop in systolic pressure, also known as the phenomenon of *pulsus paradox*. Normal pulsus paradox measures less than 12 mm Hg. [1]

Pericardial Effusion

The etiology of pericardial effusions can be vast and vary (Table 1). The most common symptoms of an effusion include fatigue, dyspnea, and chest pain. If more profound hemodynamic compromise occurs, patients may present with syncope, renal failure or shock. Those with more chronic, or subacute effusions may present with peripheral edema secondary to elevated right atrial (RA) pressure or abdominal pain from hepatic congestion.

Physical exam will reveal distended neck veins. Hemodynamically significant pleural effusions will manifest with tachycardia, arterial hypotension, and a pulsus paradox greater than 12 mm Hg. There are two other signs that are significant for pericardial effusions. Beck's triad comprises of jugular venous distention, muffled heart sounds, and hypotension. Ewart's sign depicts chronic, large pericardial effusions associated with dullness to percussion, bronchial breath sounds, and evidence of lung consolidation below the left scapula. [4]

Once an effusion is identified, the most important thing to determine is the hemodynamic sequelae, which depends vastly on the rate and volume of fluid accumulation as well as the compliance of the cardiac chambers and pericardium. A slowly expanding effusion can become quite large (>1000 mL) as the pericardial reserve volume increases. Meanwhile, a rapidly accumulating effusion can lead to marked increase in pericardial pressure with even a small volume of fluid (50 to 100 mL). [5]

Table 1. Causes of Pericardial Disease

Infectious
Bacterial (*Streptococcus, Staphylococcus, pneumococcus,* gram negative rods) Mycobacterial (tuberculosis) Viral (Coxsackie, echovirus, adenovirus, human immunodeficiency virus) Fungal (Aspergillosis, Candida, histoplasmosis) Parasitic (*Echinococcus,* amebiasis, toxoplasmosis)
Malignant
Primary mesothelioma Metastatic disease (skin, lymphoma, leukemia) Direct extension (lung cancer, breast cancer)

Metabolic
Uremia Myxedema Amyloidosis
Inflammatory
Post-myocardial infarction (Dressler's) Post-pericardiotomy syndrome Connective tissue disorders (lupus, scleroderma, polyarteritis nodosa) Sarcoidosis
Iatrogenic
Radiation induced Post-catheter based procedures Drugs (warfarin, minoxidil, procainamide)
Trauma
Blunt or penetrating chest trauma Aortic dissection Post-infarction LV rupture
Idiopathic

Cardiac Tamponade

Cardiac tamponade is a life-threatening cause of cardiogenic shock. Tamponade physiology occurs when the pressure in the pericardium exceeds the pressure in the cardiac chambers, impairing cardiac filling. [2] It is not an "all or none" phenomenon but rather a syndrome with a continuum of severity.

Echocardiography can be used to describe the hemodynamic impact of an effusion, starting with asymptomatic isolated elevation of the pericardial pressure leading up to clinical tamponade, recognized by Beck's triad. In the middle of this spectrum, echocardiography can be used to recognize tamponade by the presence of cardiac chamber collapse and alterations in respiratory variation of the mitral and tricuspid inflow pattern.

As the pressure of the pericardium continues to rise with an increase in the effusion size, the lower pressure chambers (i.e. the atria) are impaired before higher-pressure chambers (i.e. the ventricles). The ideal time to see the compressive effects of the pericardial fluid is when the pressure is lowest in the chambers, which is systole for atria and diastole for ventricles. In order to maintain cardiac output, filling pressures are elevated and tachycardia ensues. In full-blown tamponade, there is equalization of the diastolic pressures across the cardiac chambers due to the increased pericardial pressures. Any additional fluid accumulation will result in a drop in stroke volume and fall in cardiac output. [5]

It is important to note that though the coronary blood flow is reduced is tamponade, there is no ischemic component to the disease process due to the proportionally lower work load and functional requirement of the heart. [2]

Hemodynamics of Cardiac Tamponade

Cardiac tamponade continuously compresses the heart throughout the cardiac cycle, which prevents rapid atrial emptying. On echocardiography, this will be depicted as follows:

- RA systolic collapse > 1/3 systole
- RV diastolic collapse
- Reciprocal respiratory changes in ventricular volumes
- Exaggerated reciprocal respiratory changes (>25%) in ventricular filling
- Reduced early-diastolic tissue Doppler velocity
- Severe inferior vena cava dilatation

The RA free wall is a thin, flexible structure. When the intrapericardial pressure is greater than the RA systolic pressure, the RA free wall may invert or collapse even without tamponade physiology. However, if the RA free wall is inverted for a longer duration of the cycle length, then there is a greater chance of cardiac tamponade. When inversion occurs for greater than 1/3 of the cycle length, there is a 100% specificity and 94% sensitivity for the diagnosis of tamponade. [5]

If the RV free wall is normal in thickness and compliance but collapses during diastole, there is suggestion of tamponade physiology. The best view to appreciate RV diastolic collapse is the parasternal long-axis or subcostal view. RV diastolic collapse is more specific, but less sensitive than RA systolic collapse. [5]

As described earlier, there is a small inspiratory drop in systolic pressure, usually between 10-12 mmHg. With advanced phases of tamponade, this finding is exaggerated. As the right heart filling volume increases, there is a matched drop in left-sided volume, a phenomenon defined as *ventricular interdependence*.[6] On 2D imaging, tamponade physiology may be seen as *septal shifting,* which is best appreciated in the apical four-chamber view. Septal shifting occurs during inspiration with increased RV filling volume and is defined as the septal motion shifting toward the LV in diastole and toward the RV in systole. During expiration, the septal motion will normalize due to a decrease in RV volume. [5]

This pattern of septal shifting is clinically correlated with *pulsus paradoxus*. Due to augmented right heart filling during inspiration, the drop in inspiratory systolic blood pressure will exceed 12 mmHg. The hemodynamic significance of an effusion can be defined with accurate measurement of the pulsus paradox. Patients with cardiac tamponade produce a pulsus due to ventricular filling against a stiff pericardium and respiratory changes in venous pressure differential, which alternatively favor right and left ventricular filling. [3, 7]

The proper way to measure the pulsus paradox is to inflate the sphygmomanometer above the systolic blood pressure and carefully auscultating while the patient is breathing normally until the first Korotkoff sound is heard during any phase of the cardiac cycle. The first sound heart demarcates the upper limit of systolic pressure. The cuff should then continue to be slowly deflated until the Korotkoff sounds are heart with each cardiac cycle. This marks the lower limit of systolic pressures. The difference between the two is the pulsus paradox.

Other disorders that may produce a pulsus paradoxus include massive pulmonary embolism, profound hemorrhagic shock, obstructive lung disease, or other forms of severe hypotension. In contrast, the presence of RV hypertrophy, myocardial infiltrative diseases, or pulmonary hypertension may impede the identification of tamponade by making the pulsus undetectable. In addition, these conditions will obscure the classic hemodynamic findings of tamponade and patients may have a normal *y* descent on the right atrial pressure waveform despite tamponade. Other conditions that may also produce a normal pulsus paradox include atrial septal defects, severe aortic regurgitation, or elevated LV end-diastolic pressure. [1, 2, 7]

Echo Doppler recordings of RV and LV diastolic filling patterns demonstrate a similar finding to respiratory variation in ventricular volumes. With inspiration, the RV early-diastolic filling velocity will be augmented in patients with tamponade, whereas the LV diastolic filling velocity will be diminished. Differentiating the normal variation with respiration in diastolic filling from exaggerated variation (25%) as seen in tamponade patients may be difficult. [5]

With tamponade, the early-diastolic tissue Doppler velocity decreases, but returns to normal after pericardiocentesis. This is likely related to changes in cardiac output. Tamponade also results in elevated right atrial pressures, which may be seen on echocardiography as a dilated inferior vena cava with < 50% inspiratory diameter reduction.

Classic tamponade is defined as elevated and equalized right-sided diastolic pressures. With the exception of low-pressure tamponade, diastolic pressures throughout the heart are usually around 15 to 30 mmHg. Though these pressures are similar to those observed in patients with heart failure, for reasons unknown, tamponade does not produce alveolar pulmonary edema. [2, 8]

Nevertheless, there are times when low diastolic pressures (such as 6-12 mmHg) may cause serious hemodynamic compromise. This occurrence of low-pressure tamponade is thought to occur when patients are hypovolemic. A study by Sagrista-Sauleda et al analyzed the prevalence of low-pressure cardiac tamponade in patients with a pericardial effusion who also underwent careful hemodynamic studies at the time of pericardiocentesis. With their study, the authors defined low-pressure tamponade as the presence of pre-procedural intrapericardial pressure < 7 mmHg and RA pressure < 4 mmHg after intrapericardial pressure was lowered to near 0 mmHg with pericardiocentesis. Of the patients who met the hemodynamic criteria for tamponade, 20% of patients (29 of 143) had low-pressure tamponade. These patients were less likely to exhibit signs and symptoms seen with classic tamponade (24% versus 71%). [9]

Management of Tamponade

Small to moderate sized effusions do not require any treatment if there are no signs of hemodynamic compromise. Because these patients are preload dependent, it is important to prevent dehydration and avoid vasodilator drugs. In patients with hemodynamic compromise, it is important to remove the effusion. While preparing for a pericardiocentesis, hypotension can be temporized with rapid intravenous infusion of normal saline and intravenous pressor agents. [1]

The treatment of choice in unstable patients is percutaneous pericardiocentesis. If the effusion is loculated or percutaneous pericardiocentesis is not successful, surgical drainage via a pericardial window is recommended. Percutaneous balloon pericardiotomy may be utilized as a palliative measure in patients with malignant pericardial effusions to help prevent recurrence. Balloon pericardiotomy, with its percutaneous approach, has a lower mortality rate compared to pericardial windows, making it a more viable option for oncology patients. [1, 11, 12]

Pericardiocentesis may be performed at beside in a critically ill patient who is rapidly deteriorating, but it is generally performed in the cardiac catheterization laboratory. It is strongly recommended that pericardiocentesis is performed with echocardiography guidance to identify the proper site for needle insertion. With the use of 2D echocardiography, the needle may be inserted in the paraxiphoid or apical area. Without imaging, the paraxiphoid approach is recommended. In this approach, the needle is inserted between the xiphoid process and left costal margin. The needle is inserted at a 15-degree angle and is pointed toward the left shoulder. The needle should then be advanced slowly with negative pressure, until the pericardium is pierced and fluid is aspirated. [2]

A simultaneous right-heart catheterization should be performed to assess hemodynamics prior to and after fluid removal. The goal of pericardiocentesis is to attain a pericardial pressure of zero, or less. The inability to do so indicates a loculation, which requires surgical drainage. In loculated effusions, the effusion is localized by adhesions to a small area of the pericardial space. Echocardiographic evaluation from multiple acoustic windows can help reliably distinguish a loculated pericardial effusion.

After pericardiocentesis, right heart catheterization will show a decrease in right-sided diastolic pressures and the RA pressure waveforms will show a return of the *y* descent. Pericardial fluid should be sent for analysis to attempt to identify the etiology of the effusion. [1]

Constrictive Pericarditis

When the serous surfaces of the visceral and parietal pericardium become adherent, thickened, and fibrotic, the diastolic ventricular filling becomes impaired due to the loss of pericardial space. The most common causes of constrictive pericarditis are repeated episodes of pericarditis, post cardiac surgery, prior radiation exposure, connective tissue disorder, and idiopathic causes. One of the classic causes of pericardial constriction is tuberculosis. [1]

Diagnosis is often delayed due to nonspecific symptoms such as fatigue and malaise due to low cardiac output. Physical exam findings are often subtle and include elevated neck veins with a prominent *y* descent as well as distant heart sounds. Late physical exam findings include ascites and peripheral edema. Auscultation may reveal an absent apical impulse and a pericardial knock. Unlike tamponade, pulsus paradox is rare, but may be seen in cases of constrictive pericarditis with effusive constriction. [1, 5]

Physiology of Constrictive Pericarditis

With pericardial constriction, there is a reduction in pericardial space due to fibrosis, thereby reducing all cardiac chamber volume. The rigid pericardial shell limits the total volume of blood able to enter the cardiac chambers, producing competition for diastolic filling, equalization of diastolic pressures, and enhanced ventricular interdependence. In the early phase of diastole, the ventricle will rapidly fill. By mid-diastole, the predetermined volume is reached and ventricular filling is abruptly halted, causing a rapid rise in ventricular pressure. [6]

The constraining pericardium also causes an increase in ventricular interdependence. Because the pericardium is rigid, it cannot accommodate or buffer changes in the volume and pressure that occur during the cardiac and respiratory cycles. Normally, the pericardial space changes with the variations in intrathoracic pressure during respiration. Inspiration lowers intrathoracic pressure but due to the unyielding pericardium, the cardiac chamber pressure remains the same. Therefore, there will be increased venous filling into the thorax but not the right heart chambers.

Another hemodynamic response seen with pericardial constriction is diminished filling of the LV and a drop in LV systolic pressure. During inspiration, pulmonary venous pressure is lowered, however this is not transmitted to the LV. Compounded with increased ventricular interdependence, the RV filling and RV systolic pressure increase. The normal parallel fall and rise in RV and LV systolic pressure with inspiration and expiration become discordant. This discordance is highly specific and sensitive for constrictive pericarditis. [1]

Hemodynamics of Constrictive Pericarditis

Hemodynamic findings of constrictive pericarditis classically include: [1, 5]

- Elevated right-sided diastolic pressures
- *M* or *W* pattern on RA waveform with rapid fall of RA pressure with onset of ventricular filling (y descent)
- $v > a$ wave due to noncompliant RA
- Little to no respiratory variation in RA pressure
- High mid diastolic ventricular pressure plateau (*square-root* or *dip-plateau* sign)
- Failure to separate LV and RV diastolic pressures > 5 mmHg even after volume loading
- Ratio of RV end-diastolic pressure to RV systolic pressure > 1:3
- Mild elevation of RV or pulmonary artery systolic pressures (< 50 mmHg)
- Pulmonary capillary wedge pressure decline > LV early diastolic pressure during inspiration
- LV and RV systolic pressure discordance with inspiration

The RA waveform shows little respiratory variation and due to the rigid pericardium, the v wave will often be greater than the a wave since atrial contraction will be compromised by the noncompliance. The atrial pressure is increased and the ventricle is underfilled. There will be rapid right atrial emptying early in diastole with a rapid y descent on the RA waveform noted as an *M* or *W* pattern. RV filling abruptly ceases due to the constraints placed by a rigid pericardium and the ventricular waveforms may demonstrate the square root sign during diastole. [1]

It is important to note that pulmonary hypertension is rare in patients with constrictive pericarditis. RV and LV diastolic pressures are within 5 mmHg. These hemodynamic findings may be seen in other conditions. [1] (Table 2)

The most valuable hemodynamic finding associated with constrictive pericarditis is the dissociation between intrathoracic and intracardiac pressure changes with respiration. These variations can be observed in the cardiac catheterization laboratory by analyzing the pulmonary capillary wedge pressure and the LV in early diastole. Even more important is the discordance in LV and RV systolic pressures with inspiration, a sign of increased ventricular interdependence. [1]

Echocardiography is useful in differentiating tamponade and pericardial constriction in that the latter lacks effusion. Moreover, with tamponade, diastolic filling is impaired in both early and late diastole due to elevated pericardial pressures compressing the heart. In contrast, in constriction, early \diastolic filling is rapid due to the chronically underfilled state. When the predetermined volume is reached, diastolic filling will abruptly end as the limits of the rigid pericardial space are attained. [1] In addition, constrictive disease states will demonstrate > 25% drop in mitral inflow during inspiration. Hepatic vein flow will be reversed during expiration. [6]

Other imaging modalities such as chest computed tomography (CT) and magnetic resonance imaging (MRI) may also be useful in diagnosing constrictive pericarditis by demonstrating pericardial thickening. [6] A minority of cases may also reveal pericardial calcification on chest X-ray or fluoroscopy.[5]

Management of Constrictive Pericarditis

If patients are mildly symptomatic and have relatively low RA pressures, they may be treated medically with diuretics. These patients should be followed with reassessment of the RA pressure. A significant number of patients with constrictive pericarditis will require surgical pericardiectomy to effectively lower RA pressure and improve symptoms. [1] In patients with evidence of ongoing pericardial inflammation, a course of anti-inflammatory therapy with NSAIDs, colchicine, or corticosteroids may be utilized first to treat the inflammatory process without requiring surgery. [6]

Effusive-Constrictive Pericarditis

Patients with pericarditis who continue to have hemodynamic abnormalities with persistent RA pressure elevation despite removal of all pericardial fluid may have a continued pericardial abnormality, usually secondary to inflammation and a constricting effect of the visceral pericardium. In these patients, the RA waveform will be prominent and there will be a rapid *y* descent similar to patients with constriction. This entity is coined as effusive-constrictive pericarditis, which is rare, but found in 8% of tamponade patients who have undergone cardiac catheterization. [2, 10]

Generally, these patients will have a constrictive component that improves as the inflammatory process subsides, but some patients may have chronic constriction and will require pericardiectomy.

Table 2. Causes of Constrictive Physiology (Pseudoconstriction)

Restrictive cardiomyopathy
RV infarction
Pulmonary hypertension
Obesity
Severe tricuspid regurgitation
Acute volume overload
Acute heart failure
Acute severe mitral regurgitation

Restrictive Cardiomyopathy

Restrictive cardiomyopathy is used to describe a group of uncommon disorders with impaired ventricular filling in the setting of preserved ventricular systolic function. With increased ventricular stiffness, the ventricles become noncompliant causing elevated pressures during diastole and only a small increase in ventricular volumes.

Some of the most common etiologies of restrictive cardiomyopathy include endomyocardial fibrosis, amyloidosis, and idiopathic restrictive cardiomyopathy. Differentiating between constrictive pericarditis and restrictive cardiomyopathy is difficult due to the similar nature of clinical presentation and hemodynamic abnormalities. Pericardial thickening may also be difficult to appreciate. [1, 5]

Other features that favor restrictive pericarditis include:

- Separation of ventricular diastolic pressures of more than 5 mmHg
- Ratio of RV end-diastolic pressure to RV systolic pressure < 1:3
- Moderate to severe elevation of RV or pulmonary artery systolic pressures (>50 mmHg)

The discordance in RV and LV systolic pressures during inspiration remains as one of the most valuable means of differentiating constrictive pericarditis and restrictive cardiomyopathy. Other clinical features more consistent with restriction include biatrial enlargement and aortic valve regurgitation. ECG abnormalities such as low voltage and conduction delays may also be seen in patients with restrictive cardiomyopathy. Restrictive cardiomyopathy has also been seen to elevate levels of B-type natriuretic peptide compared to the normal levels seen in constriction. [13] B-type natriuretic peptide levels vary directly with ventricular wall stress and are likely less elevated in constriction due to the limits imposed on ventricular stretch by the constraining pericardium. If restrictive cardiomyopathy is suspected, endomyocardial biopsy may be considered to assist in obtaining a diagnosis.

Features that favor constriction include pericardial calcification and thickened pericardium, which may be seen on CT or MRI. There is also the possibility that restrictive cardiomyopathy and constrictive pericarditis coexist. This duality of syndromes is seen in patients with sarcoidosis, those with prior radiation exposure, and in those with hypereosinophilic syndrome. [1]

References

[1] Ragosta, R. Pericardial Disease and Restrictive Cardiomyopathy. *Textbook of Clinical Hemodynamics*. 1st Edition, 2008, 123-147.

[2] Spodick, D. Acute Cardiac Tamponade. *New England Journal of Medicine*, 2003, 349, 684-690.

[3] Reddy, PS; Curtiss, EI; et al. Cardiac Tamponade: Hemodynamic Observations in Man. *Circulation*, 1978, 58, 265-272

[4] Ewart, W. Practical Aids in the Diagnosis of Pericardial Effusion, in Connection with the Question as to Surgical Treatment. *The British Medical Journal*, 1896, 1, 717-721.

[5] Otto, C. Pericardial Disease. *Textbook of Clinical Echocardiography.* 5th Edition, 2013, 254-270.

[6] Borlaug, B. Pericardial Diseases. *ACCSAP 8*, 2012, 18.1.1-18.1.8.

[7] Swami, A; Spodick, DH. Pulsus Paradoxus in Cardiac Tamponade: A Pathophysiologic Continuum. *Clinical Cardiology*, 2003, 26, 215-217.

[8] Antman, EM; Cargill, V; Grossman, W. Low-Pressure Cardiac Tamponade. *Annals of Internal Medicine*, 1979, 91, 403-406.

[9] Sagristà-Sauleda, J; Angel, J; Sambola, A; et al. Low-Pressure Cardiac Tamponade. Clinical and Hemodynamic Profile. *Circulation*, 2006, 113, 945-952.

[10] Sagristà-Sauleda, J; Angel, J; Sánchez, A; et al. Effusive-constrictive pericarditis. *New England Journal of Medicine*, 2004, 350, 469-475.

[11] Ziskind, AA; Pearce, AC; Lemmon, CC; et al. Percutaneous Balloon Pericardiotomy for the Treatment of Cardiac Tamponade and Large Pericardial Effusions: Description of Technique and Report of the First 50 Cases. *Journal of American College of Cardiology*, 1993, 21, 1-5.

[12] Puril, A; Agarwal, N; Dwivedi, SK; et al. Percutaneous balloon pericardiotomy for the treatment of recurrent malignant pericardial effusion. *Indian Heart Journal*, 2012, Jan, 64 (1), 88-89.

[13] Leya, FS; Arab, D; et al. The efficacy of brain natriuretic peptide levels in differentiating constrictive pericarditis from restrictive cardiomyopathy. *Journal of American College of Cardiology*, 2005, 45, 1900–1902.

In: Cardiac Tamponade
Editor: Cameron L. Pittman

ISBN: 978-1-63482-787-4

Chapter 3

Lactate Metabolism and Tissue Perfusion in Cardiac Tamponade: Lesson Learned from Experimental Models

José Gorrasi
Departamento de Medicina Intensiva, Centro Asistencial Sindicato Médico del Uruguay (CASMU), Montevideo, Uruguay

Abstract

Cardiac tamponade (CT) is a life-threatening clinical syndrome that requires timely diagnosis. CT is defined as a haemodynamically significant cardiac compression caused by pericardial fluid. The fluid may be blood, pus, effusion (transudate or exudate) or air and treatment involves correction of the cardiac diastolic restriction by removing pericardial fluid during either pericardiocentesis or thoracotomy.

In CT systemic arterial hypoperfusion is followed by regional blood flow redistribution in order to preserve tissue and organ function. In this chapter we reviewed regional blood flow and metabolic derangements reported in experimental models. In the early stages of CT Portal venous flow reduction is associated with an increase in hepatic arterial blood flow, whereas in the late stage of low blood flow total hepatic blood flow is decreased despite redistribution between portal venous and hepatic arterial blood flow. The preservation of liver blood flow is due to a regulatory mechanism known as the hepatic artery buffer response (HABR).

In CT there are profound changes in the regional oxygen metabolism. Hepatic oxygen extraction reached values around 80%. Portal oxygen content became low due to an increase in mesenteric oxygen extraction during systemic low blood flow.

Accordingly, in conditions of low portal blood flow, the HABR and redistribution of blood flow in the celiac trunk become critical for the maintenance of sufficient hepatic oxygen delivery. CT induces inadequate visceral perfusion which may interfere with integrity of the intestinal mucosal barrier and contribute to the development of multiple organ dysfunction. Gut luminal lactate increased relatively late during low systemic blood flow and could be explained by systemic hyperlactatemia. The proportional blood flow of the superior mesenteric artery was well maintained during progressive, severe CT and signs of systemic hypoperfusion preceded those of gut hypoperfusion. Signs of gut hypoperfusion (increased veno-arterial and mucosal arterial PCO_2 gradients as well as increased regional CO_2 content difference) preceded the signs of inadequate mucosal oxygen supply and the signs of gross jejunal wall dysoxia.

Arterial blood lactate increased early during tamponade and was not explained by increased gut lactate release. Systemic hyperlactatemia is apparently due to lactate release from other tissues than the gut, but is also partly caused by decreasing hepatic clearance. Changes in lactate metabolism are not related to cell injury since Hepatic lactate extraction decreased, but hepatic release of glutathione Stransferase A did not change during CT. During low systemic perfusion, the HABR is exhausted and hepatic function is impaired without signs of cellular damage. Whole body venous efflux as an estimate of hepatic and extra-hepatic organ lactate efflux is of similar magnitude in hyperdynamic sepsis and in cardiogenic shock. In cardiac tamponade, regional, extra-splanchnic lactate production is accompanied by hepatic failure to increase oxygen extraction and net hepatic lactate output, despite maintained hepatic arterial perfusion. After CT it has been reported that vascular dysfunction persisted up to 6 h after release of tamponade. These inflammatory characteristics may also indicate that inflammatory activation is a possible pathway involved in the pathogenesis of cardiogenic shock. In a porcine model of acute splanchnic hypoperfusion, endothelin blockade restored hepato mesenteric perfusion and reversed lactate metabolism. These observations might be relevant when considering liver protection in low CO states.

Coronary Regional Blood Flow and Cardiac Tamponade

It is known that coronary artery blood flow decreases and cardiac work decreased during CT. In a model of CT in conscious dogs CT causes a decline in coronary artery blood flow and increase in myocardial oxygen extraction, in this phase of CT the lactate-pyruvate ratio did not change, and there was no evidence of myocardial lactate production [1]. Crystal et al[2] assess myocardial and systemic responses to CT alone and combined with arterial hypoxemia in dog model of CT. Myocardial regional blood flow and lactate extraction were assessed. CT decreases myocardial regional blood flow and myocardial VO_2 but had no effect on myocardial lactate extraction. Regional blood flow decreased in kidney, splanchnic organs, skeletal muscle, and skin, but it had no effect in brain. The regulatory vasodilator mechanisms that occur during combined CT and hypoxia, were capable of maintaining adequate oxygen supply in myocardium and brain but not apparently in the non vital tissues where these mechanisms were antagonized by reflex vasoconstriction. Volume challenge is part of resuscitation therapies in the early phases of shock. When implemented in experimental models of shock, volume resuscitation after CT did not recovered stroke volume, coronary sinus pressure and coronary perfusion pressure. As a result these results shown that CT neither produce myocardial ischemia nor increase lactate production but impairs coronary hemodynamics. There were no recovery in coronary perfusion pressure after initial treatment such as volume resuscitation [3].

Complex surgical procedures during CT could associate systemic low blood flow especially during anesthesia induction. Crystal et al. tested the hypothesis that the anesthetic technique will influence the changes in regional blood flow during intraoperative CT. CT causes a decrease in regional blood flow that were similar with different anesthetic drugs (ketamine, fentanyl or midazolam and isoflurane) used, except for regional blood flow in subcortical regions of the brain and in the spinal cord were maintained under isoflurane but decreased under ketamine or midazolam. Due to regional regulatory mechanisms that counterbalanced decrease in regional blood flow no significant metabolic changes occurs [4].

Lactate Metabolism in Cardiac Tamponade

Systemic low blood flow state leads to regional blood flow redistribution, and modifications in VO_2/DO_2 relationships. When anaerobic threshold is present anaerobic metabolism and lactate production occurs. Lactate origin in shock may be associated with anaerobic metabolism or inflammatory production due to other mechanisms than hypoxia. The lactate production and clearance during shock was evaluated in a model of CT by using a constant infusion of 14C-labeled lactate, the percentage of lactate undergoing oxidation and the total carbon dioxide production from lactate was evaluated. Shock was induced by hemorrhage, CT, and endotoxin. In shock there were an increase of lactate concentration and lactate turnover, while lactate turnover decreased. The percentage of lactate oxidation remained normal whereas the percentage of CO_2 derived from lactate increased. Since VO_2 and CO_2 remained unchanged, this is associated with increased metabolism of substrates that used lactate and pyruvate as intermediate substrates such as carbohydrates and amino acids instead of substrates that not form pyruvate that is free fatty acids. Then, during shock elevated arterial lactate in shock was due to an increase in the lactate production and not to a lack of tisular oxygen or hypoxia [5-7].

Cilley et al., evaluated the effect of low oxygen delivery produced by anemia, hypoxia, and low cardiac output in pentobarbital-anesthetized dogs[8]. Oxygen delivery was decreased by isovolemic dilutional anemia, breathing hypoxic gas mixtures, or CT. Below the critical level of oxygen delivery (DO_2crit), VO_2 fell (became supply dependent) and lactic acidosis occurred, regardless of the mechanism of impaired oxygen delivery. Tissue hypoxia may be relevant in hyperlactatemia during sepsis or endotoxemic shock. CT is a useful experimental model to study the effects of decreasing DO_2 to a critical level where anaerobic metabolism starts. The effects of endotoxin on the oxygen extraction capabilities of the body during CT were studied in experimental CT. DO_2 was reduced up to critical DO_2 delivery by CT and critical oxygen extraction and lactate concentration were measured. In CT the mixed venous PO_2 levels at DO_2crit were higher in the endotoxic than in CT alone. Arterial blood lactate concentration was higher in the endotoxic than in the CT alone [9].

It has been reported that increases in veno arterial difference in PCO_2 and arteriovenous difference in pH are valuable markers of tissue hypoxia in shock states associated with low CO. The relationship between of veno arterial difference in PCO_2 and arteriovenous difference in pH and lactate with VO_2 and DO_2 in CT was evaluated in a model of CT with reduction of blood flow up to critical DO_2. When DO_2 was reduced in a stepwise manner veno arterial difference in PCO_2 and arteriovenous difference in pH and lactate increased significantly up to critical DO_2 and this increase was more pronounced below this level. Arterial lacate concentration was associated with arterial hypocapnia and mixed venous hypercapnia[10].

Hyperlactatemia in shock is due to several mechanisms including aerobic stimulation of sodium ATPasa and glycolisis stimulation [11, 12]. Beta adrenergic drugs increase aerobic lactate production by glycolisis rate enhancement [11]. Since Lactate production is influenced by vasoactive drugs used in shock states, particularly cardiogenic shock. In a model of CT with decrease in blood flow below critical level of DO_2, the use of dobutamine and norepinephrine increased CO and DO_2. VO_2 at critical DO_2 was high with dobutamine and critical pericardial pressure was higher in dobutamine treated animals than in control group. At critical DO_2, blood lactate concentration was lower in the dobutamine-treated animals than in controls. In CT, Dobutamine delayed the onset of tissue hypoxia by increasing blood flow and oxygen availability and decrease lactate production [13]. This is in concordance with the findings that isoproterenol increased macrohemodynamics and microhemodynamics and liver and gut oxygen extraction capabilities. Increase capillary density and increased capillary perfusion is related in part to localyl adenosine monophosphate release. Isoproterenol increased lactate and decrease arterial pH as a result of increased glycolysis [14].

During low blood flow states oxygen free radicals are produced by several mechanisms, on the other hand after treatment and reperfusion there are mechanisms that increase oxygen free radical production and potentiate endothelial cell damage. Because oxygen free radical production modulation is a potential treatment for reperfusion injury this was investigated in experimental models that combine CT with endotoxin in order to evaluate oxygen extraction capabilities. N-acetyl-L-cysteine (NAC) a thiol provider and free radical scavenger was evaluated in a combined model of endotoxin and CT. After CT critical DO_2 was lower in NAC group (endotoxin + CT without NAC), and critical EO_2R and the slope of depend part of the VO_2/DO_2 relationship was higher in the NAC group compared to control group (endotoxin + CT without NAC). Accordingly, lactate concentration and TNF production were lower in the NAC group meaning that there was a modulation of oxidative stress in part due to NAC and glutathione peroxidase, an enzyme that uses thiols groups provided by NAC [13]. Macrohemodynamics variables were also high in the NAC group suggesting a vascular and myocardial effect of NAC. A similar pattern was observed with the antioxidant 21-aminosteroid

U-74006F [15] in a endotoxin and CT experimental model. The antioxidant decreased critical DO_2 and increased critical EO_2R, meanwhile systemic and regional lactate were lower in treated animals suggesting a protective effect and a link between lactate production and oxidative stress.

Hypoxantine, Xanthine and Adenosine are produced during persistent low blood flow states as a result of low oxygen supply that triggers nucleotide catabolism. Adenosine induces local vasodilatation by adenosine receptor stimulation and increases regional O_2 availability and extraction. In a model of endotoxin and CT the nucleoside transport inhibitor draflazine (that increases extracellular adenosine by blocking adenosine uptake from extracellular space) modifies the O_2 extraction capabilities differently, in liver it decreases critical DO_2 and it increases liver critical EO_2R whereas in gut it increases critical DO_2. As a result draflazine delayed O_2 supply dependence in liver but not in gut. Draftlazine decrease ileal mucosal perfusion and renal artery blood flow. On the other hand, hepatic artery blood flow, mesenteric artery blood flow, portal vein blood flow and liver perfusion were not modified by draflazine. Portal and hepatic lactate tent to be lower in treated animals (although non significant), suggesting less hepatosplanchnic ischemia than in endotoxin plus CT not treated group [16]. Tumor necrosis factor increase lately in this model of CT (after 190 min) suggesting that adenosine transport inhibitor may modulate tumor necrosis turnover (figure 1).

The role of the hepatosplanchic area in the contribution to hyperlactatemia in sepsis was evaluated with a model that combines endoxin infusion and tissue ischemia induced by CT [17]. It is well known that high blood lactate concentrations over re associated with a poor clinical outcome [18-21]. Hepatosplanchnic lactate release could be due to increased lactate gut production, decreased clearance or both. In low blood flow tissue hypoxia is the main factor in lactate production. In a model of endotoxin alone and endotoxin followed by endotoxin and CT hepatosplanchnic lactate production was evaluated. After 30 minutes of endoxin infusion the gut shift from lactate consumer to a lactate producer, liver lactate uptake increase with no changes in liver lactate extraction and hepatosplachnic lactate production. When CT was added to endotoxin liver lactate uptake and liver lactate extraction decreased and became negative (lactate is released from liver). Gut lactate production remain positive but in endotoxin plus CT group there was a significant decrease in gut lactate production. Hepatosplanchnic lactate production was significant different between endotoxin and endotoxin plus CT from 90 minutes to 180 minutes and became positive (lactate producer) after 120 minutes of CT plus endotoxin.

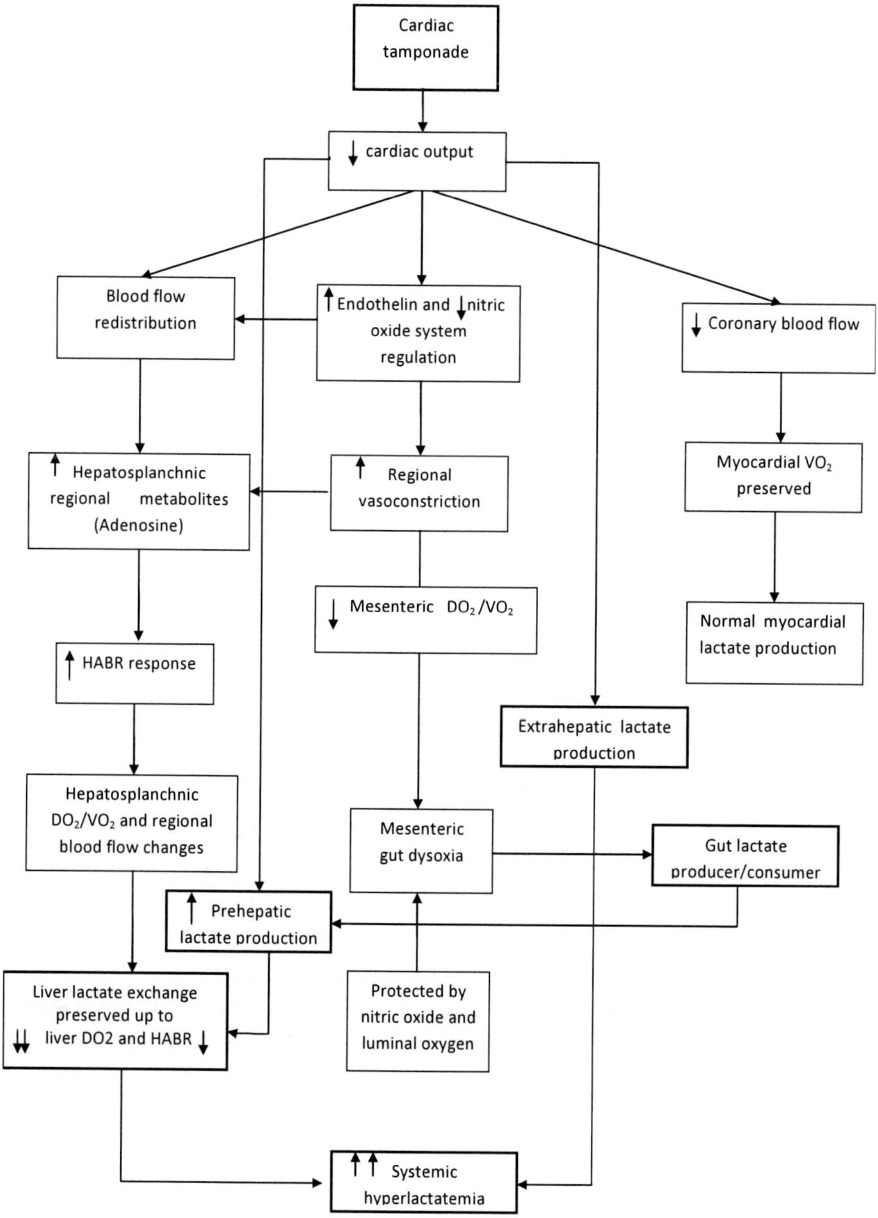

Figure 1.

Gut lactate production remain positive in both groups, but decreases in CT along the experiment, mainly due to a decrease in portal venous flow. When liver lactate extraction and hepatosplanchnic lactate production were analyzed together oxygen transport by plotting against liver DO_2 divided critical liver DO_2 for each dog (when this relationship is below 1 there is supply-dependent oxygen metabolism when is above 1 there is no dependency) liver lactate became negative and hepatosplanchnic lactate production became positive when liver DO_2 falls below its critical level. This is in agreement with experimental model of CT that evaluated the differential contribution of splanchnic organs to hyperlactatemia in CT or in peritonitis [22]. Septic and cardiogenic shock has different effects on hepatosplanchnic lactate exchange and systemic hyperlactatemia. Hepatic lactate influx increased in peritonitis and in CT, hepatic lactate uptake remained unchanged in peritonitis and decreased in CT. The contribution of Hepatic lactate efflux to whole body venous efflux was higher in CT than in peritonitis (mixed venous lactate concentration multiplied by CO). Whole body venous lactate efflux (an estimate of hepatic and extra-hepatic organ lactate efflux) is of similar magnitude in peritonitis and CT, but, changes in arterial lactate over time were due to different mechanisms [22]. In peritonitis, whole body venous efflux increased early, due to extra-splanchnic, extra-renal lactate production, and the liver lactate uptake was preserved (liver is a lactate consumer). In contrast, in CT, extra-splanchnic lactate production increased and the hepatic lactate uptake reverted to net hepatic lactate efflux (liver became a producer). The net hepatic lactate output was associated with a failure of increase in hepatic oxygen extraction. Hepatic arterial perfusion was preserved, but portal venous blood flow and oxygen content decreased markedly. In this model unchanged regional pCO_2 gradients and maintained regional oxygen consumption suggest that increased glycolysis rather than tissue hypoxia was the cause of increased lactate efflux (figure 1).

It has been demonstrated that hepatic lactate uptake can increase acutely by several fold, if hepatic perfusion is preserved [23]. The failure of hepatic lactate uptake to increase in CT is likely explained (like in the endotoxin plus tamponade study) by the decrease of hepatic perfusion and oxygen delivery below a critical level. In CT, the increased central venous pressures reduced the hepatic blood flow more than in cardiogenic shock caused by other mechanisms. Venous lactate efflux from the systemic circulation was of a similar magnitude in peritonitis and in severe cardiogenic shock. In peritonitis, this was the consequence of an early increase in peripheral, extra-splanchnic, extra-renal lactate production without signs of tissue hypoxia but impaired capability to increase hepatic lactate uptake. In cardiogenic shock, the increased venous lactate efflux was the result of increased net lactate release from both the periphery and from the liver [22]. In CT, regional, extra-splanchnic lactate production is accompanied by hepatic failure to increase oxygen extraction and net hepatic lactate output, despite maintained hepatic arterial perfusion. Hepatic lactate uptake (hepatic lactate influx – hepatic lactate efflux) decreases when CO was severely reduced suggesting that liver lactate metabolism is altered when liver perfusion is critically reduced and the HABR exhausted. No cellular damage was observed in the liver enzyme profile [24]. CT induces a systemic decrease in blood flow that leads to hepatosplanchnic low blood flow and regional oxygen metabolism changes. Compared with other mechanisms of blood flow impairment such as mesenteric ischemia and isolated regional blood flow reduction in CT shown a regional decrease in all blood flows except for hepatic artery blood flow that is preserved and increased until severe CT occurs, this is associated with liver DO_2 and gut DO_2 decrease and liver ERO_2 and gut ERO_2 increase. Hepatic artery buffer response helped to maintain hepatic oxygen extraction and consumption during regional low blood flow (figure 1) [25].

In CT gut luminal lactate production may be a marker of cellular dysoxia following critical systemic blood flow reduction. Experimental models have shown that gut luminal lactate increased lately and it is explained by systemic arterial hyperlactatemia. Superior mesenteric blood flow is preserved and signs of systemic hypoperfusion preceded signs of gut hypoperfusion (veno arterial PCO_2 gradients, mucosal to arterial PCO_2 gradients, regional PCO_2 differences), that are followed by signs of cellular jejunum wall dysoxia expressed by gut luminal lactate release and mesenteric ketone body ratio alterations. This is in concordance with the above studies where liver lactate production occurs late and after a profound reduction in hepatosplanchnic blood flow. Gut luminal lactate concentration was explained by mucosal epithelial release of lactate, diffusion of lactate from subepithelial mucosa from arterial blood flow and capillaries and epithelial uptake of lactate with arterial lactate overload from extra-splanchnic tissues (figure 1) [26].

Effect of Experimental Treatment on Regional Blood Flow and Metabolism

Volume expansion and fluid resuscitation is used in shock states in order to improve peripheral circulation and regional perfusion. The effect of volume expansion was evaluated in CT models. Van Genderen et al., studied the regional perfusion during experimental endotoxemic and obstructive shock by CT and compare the effect of initial CO-targeted fluid resuscitation with optimal CO-targeted resuscitation on regional perfusion on different peripheral tissues [27]. Changes were similar but endotoxemic sepsis displayed greater regional perfusion heterogeneity [28]. The effects of Hypertonic saline-dextran on cardiac performance and splanchnic perfusion were evaluate in experimental CT [29]. Resuscitation with Hypertonic saline-dextran restored portal venous blood flow, and improved gastric, jejunal, hepatic and renal microcirculation, this improvement was maintained following release of CT. There were no signs of cardiac depression. Since hypertonic colloid solutions could be protective on the microcirculation the effects of hypertonic saline hydroxyl ethyl starch were compared with isotonic saline solution in endotoxin sepsis followed by CT to evaluated oxygen transport and extraction after resuscitation. When CT was induced to study the tissue oxygen extraction capabilities, hypertonic saline hypertonic saline hydroxyl ethyl starch -treated had a lower critical oxygen delivery, and a significantly higher critical oxygen extraction ratio than the isotonic group. Hypertonic saline hydroxyl ethyl starch solution can increase whole body oxygen extraction capabilities, by an improvement in microvascular perfusion in septic conditions[30]. During CT, intravascular volume expansion increased CO only in animals which were initially volume-depleted. Volume expansion of normovolemic or hypervolemic animals caused minimal changes in CO, but increased atrial and aortic pressures [31].

Regional Vasoconstrictor Systems and Nitric Oxide during Cardiac Tamponade

The renin angiotensin system is involved y vascular tone regulation and blood volume homeostasis, when a critical blood flow reduction is present renin is released from kidneys in order to preserve blood volume homeostasis. The role of the renin angiotensin axis in cardiogenic shock was evaluated in an experimental CT model. During CT there was a disproportionate decrease in mesenteric blood flow with similar increase in mesenteric vascular resistance. Prior blockade of the renin angiontensin system eliminated the contribution of mesenteric vascular resistance to the systemic vascular resistance while alpha blockade has no effect. Then, rennin angiotensin system mediated selective mesenteric vasoconstriction and increased systemic vascular resistance in cardiogenic shock [32].

Acute decrease in systemic blood flow are associated with redistribution of blood flow away from splanchnic region. Regional vasoconstrictors are involved in this response, endothelin molecule that is more potent vasoconstrictor than norepinephinre. In experimental CT the use of iloporost vasodilates mesenteric artery, reversed gut hypercarbia without systemic changes in CO or mean arterial pressure l. [33]. The combined ET_A–ET_B receptor antagonist tezosentan administered after CT normalize portal venous blood flow, hepatic and mesenteric oxygen delivery and extraction without changes on CO or hepatic blood flow. Hepatic and mesenteric handling of lactate was converted to extraction [34]. The combined ET_A–ET_B antagonist tezosentan restored portal venous blood flow and laser Doppler flowmetry to baseline values, and decreased PCO_2 gaps. Restored mucosal blood flow and oxygenation, are important for mucosal barrier integrity [35]. Snygg et al., found that of Jejunal nitric oxide (NO) formation is impaired during jejunal mucosal hypoperfusion. Mesenteric hypoperfusion was induced by CT, this was associated with decreases in jejuna NO formation, mesenteric oxygen delivery, oxygen consumption and delivery. Jejunal NO production was not restored after jejunal lumen perfusion with L-arginine whereas jejunal lumen perfusion with oxygen restored jejunal NO levels. Therefore oxygen rather than L-arginine is the limiting factor in NO production during reduced splanchic blood flow by CT [36]

Inflammatory Response in Cardiac Tamponade

Besides cellular injury due to tissue hypoxia and anaerobic metabolism, low blood flow states could induce inflammation by several mechanisms. Moreover, the persistence of these alterations once macrohemodynamics is restored may influence clinical outcome and multiple organ failure. During the recovery phase of CT inflammatory characteristics such as high temperature and interleukin-6 were present. It has been reported that vascular dysfunction and cardiac dysfunction persist up to 6 hours after release of CT [37]. High levels of cardiac troponin T, vasoactive inflammatory mediators, including histamine, nitrite/nitrate, big-endothelin, superoxide and high-mobility group box protein-1 were observed in a model of CT after tamponade release [38].

This was associated with intestinal leukocyte and complement activation. Splanchnic macro- and microcirculatory complications in cardiogenic shock are linked to local and systemic inflammatory activation. The administration of a C5 complement inhibitor (acetyl-peptide-A) restored mean arterial pressure and CO, while the plasma superoxide, high-mobility group box protein-1, big-endothelin, and intestinal myeloperoxidase levels were reduced suggesting a protective effect of complement activation modulation [39] . In a model of sepsis in wich CT was used to study the DO_2-VO_2 relationship, the use of interleukin–1beta [40] impairs oxygen extraction even before VO_2 becomes supply-dependent.

Regional Blood Flow and Lactate Production in Cardiac Tamponade

Respiratory muscle lactate production during low blood flow could be associated with poor outcome. The respiratory muscle blood flow and organ blood flow was evaluated in dogs with CT divided to mechanical ventilation and muscle paralysis and to spontaneous breathing. After 50 min of CT, blood flow to the respiratory muscles increased during tamponade in spontaneously breathing (diaphragmatic flow increased to 361%), while it decreased in mechanically ventilated. Spontaneonus breathing when systemic blood flow is reduced or when metabolic demands are increased could explain tissue ischemia in non respiratory organs. In spontaneously breathing the respiratory muscles received 21% of the CO, compared with only 3% in the mechanically ventilated group. Mechanical ventilation unload respiratory work and decrease metabolic demands. As a result the percentage of CO toward diaphragm is reduced. Blood flows to the liver, brain, and quadriceps muscles were higher in CT in the mechanically ventilated group but not in spontaneously breathing animals. Respiratory muscles were the main source of arterial lactate in respiratory distress and fatigue. This is reversed after intubation and mechanical ventilation. Blood lactate at after the induction CT was lower in the mechanically ventilated group [41].

References

[1] Klopfenstein HS, Bernath GA, Cogswell TL, Boerboom LE: Coronary artery hemodynamics in conscious dog during cardiac tamponade. *Circ Res* 1987, 60(6):845-849.

[2] Crystal GJ, Salem MR: Myocardial and systemic responses to arterial hypoxemia during cardiac tamponade. *Am J Physiol* 1989, 257(3 Pt 2):H726-733.

[3] Johnston WE, Vinten-Johansen J, McGivor AC, Santamore WP, Block SM, Moulton KP: Efficacy of intravascular volume resuscitation in dogs with acute cardiac tamponade. *Ann Thorac Surg* 1988, 45(6):667-673.

[4] Crystal GJ, Metwally AA, Salem MR: Isoflurane preserves central nervous system blood flow during intraoperative cardiac tamponade in dogs. *Can J Anaesth* 2004, 51(10):1011-1017.

[5] Daniel AM, Pierce CH, MacLean LD, Shizgal HM: Lactate metabolism in the dog during shock from hemorrhage, cardiac tamponade or endotoxin. *Surg Gynecol Obstet* 1976, 143(4):581-586.

[6] Daniel AM, Pierce CH, Shizgal HM, MacLean LD: Lactate turnover in oligemic and normovolemic shock. *Surg Forum* 1974, 25(0):3-4.

[7] Daniel AM, Shizgal HM, MacLean LD: The anatomic and metabolic source of lactate in shock. *Surg Gynecol Obstet* 1978, 147(5):697-700.

[8] Cilley RE, Scharenberg AM, Bongiorno PF, Guire KE, Bartlett RH: Low oxygen delivery produced by anemia, hypoxia, and low cardiac output. *J Surg Res* 1991, 51(5):425-433.

[9] Zhang H, Vincent JL: Oxygen extraction is altered by endotoxin during tamponade-induced stagnant hypoxia in the dog. *Circ Shock* 1993, 40(3):168-176.

[10] Zhang H, Vincent JL: Arteriovenous differences in PCO2 and pH are good indicators of critical hypoperfusion. *Am Rev Respir Dis* 1993, 148(4 Pt 1):867-871.

[11] Levy B, Gibot S, Franck P, Cravoisy A, Bollaert PE: Relation between muscle Na+K+ ATPase activity and raised lactate concentrations in septic shock: a prospective study. *Lancet* 2005, 365(9462):871-875.

[12] James JH, Fang CH, Schrantz SJ, Hasselgren PO, Paul RJ, Fischer JE: Linkage of aerobic glycolysis to sodium-potassium transport in rat skeletal muscle. Implications for increased muscle lactate production in sepsis. *J Clin Invest* 1996, 98(10):2388-2397.

[13] Zhang H, Spapen H, Nguyen DN, Benlabed M, Buurman WA, Vincent JL: Protective effects of N-acetyl-L-cysteine in endotoxemia. *Am J Physiol* 1994, 266(5 Pt 2):H1746-1754.

[14] Zhang H, De Jongh R, De Backer D, Cherkaoui S, Vray B, Vincent JL: Effects of alpha - and beta -adrenergic stimulation on hepatosplanchnic perfusion and oxygen extraction in endotoxic shock. *Crit Care Med* 2001, 29(3):581-588.

[15] Zhang H, Spapen H, Manikis P, Rogiers P, Metz G, Buurman WA, Vincent JL: Tirilazad mesylate (U-74006F) inhibits effects of endotoxin in dogs. *Am J Physiol* 1995, 268(5 Pt 2):H1847-1855.

[16] Zhang H, De Jongh R, Cherkaoui S, Shahram M, Vray B, Vincent JL: Effects of nucleoside transport inhibition on hepatosplanchnic perfusion, oxygen extraction capabilities, and TNF release during acute endotoxic shock. *Shock* 2001, 15(5):378-385.

[17] Creteur J, De Backer D, Sun Q, Vincent JL: The hepatosplanchnic contribution to hyperlactatemia in endotoxic shock: effects of tissue ischemia. *Shock* 2004, 21(5):438-443.

[18] Bakker J, Coffernils M, Leon M, Gris P, Vincent JL: Blood lactate levels are superior to oxygen-derived variables in predicting outcome in human septic shock. *Chest* 1991, 99(4):956-962.

[19] Bernardin G, Pradier C, Tiger F, Deloffre P, Mattei M: Blood pressure and arterial lactate level are early indicators of short-term survival in human septic shock. *Intensive Care Med* 1996, 22(1):17-25.

[20] Marecaux G, Pinsky MR, Dupont E, Kahn RJ, Vincent JL: Blood lactate levels are better prognostic indicators than TNF and IL-6 levels in patients with septic shock. *Intensive Care Med* 1996, 22(5):404-408.

[21] Bellomo R, Kellum JA, Pinsky MR: Transvisceral lactate fluxes during early endotoxemia. *Chest* 1996, 110(1):198-204.

[22] Gorrasi J, Eleftheriadis A, Takala J, Brandt S, Djafarzadeh S, Bruegger LE, Bracht H, Jakob SM: Different contribution of splanchnic organs to hyperlactatemia in fecal peritonitis and cardiac tamponade. *Biomed Res Int* 2013, 2013:251084.

[23] Jakob SM, Merasto-Minkkinen M, Tenhunen JJ, Heino A, Alhava E, Takala J: Prevention of systemic hyperlactatemia during splanchnic ischemia. *Shock* 2000, 14(2):123-127.

[24] Jakob SM, Tenhunen JJ, Laitinen S, Heino A, Alhava E, Takala J: Effects of systemic arterial hypoperfusion on splanchnic hemodynamics and hepatic arterial buffer response in pigs. *Am J Physiol Gastrointest Liver Physiol* 2001, 280(5):G819-827.

[25] Bracht H, Takala J, Tenhunen JJ, Brander L, Knuesel R, Merasto-Minkkinen M, Jakob SM: Hepatosplanchnic blood flow control and oxygen extraction are modified by the underlying mechanism of impaired perfusion. *Crit Care Med* 2005, 33(3):645-653.

[26] Tenhunen JJ, Jakob S, Ruokonen E, Takala J: Jejunal luminal microdialysate lactate in cardiac tamponade--effect of low systemic blood flow on gut mucosa. *Intensive Care Med* 2002, 28(7):953-962.

[27] van Genderen ME, Paauwe J, de Jonge J, van der Valk RJ, Lima A, Bakker J, van Bommel J: Clinical assessment of peripheral perfusion to predict postoperative complications after major abdominal surgery early: a prospective observational study in adults. *Crit Care* 2014, 18(3):R114.

[28] van Genderen ME, Klijn E, Lima A, de Jonge J, Sleeswijk Visser S, Voorbeijtel J, Bakker J, van Bommel J: Microvascular perfusion as a target for fluid resuscitation in experimental circulatory shock. *Crit Care Med* 2014, 42(2):e96-e105.

[29] Terajima K, Aneman A, Haljamae H: Haemodynamic effects of volume resuscitation by hypertonic saline-dextran (HSD) in porcine acute cardiac tamponade. *Acta Anaesthesiol Scand* 2004, 48(1):46-54.

[30] Maciel F, Mook M, Zhang H, Vincent JL: Comparison of hypertonic with isotonic saline hydroxyethyl starch solution on oxygen extraction capabilities during endotoxic shock. *Shock* 1998, 9(1):33-39.

[31] Grose R, Greenberg MA, Yipintsoi T, Cohen MV: Cardiac tamponade in dogs with normal coronary arteries. I. Effect of changing intravascular volume on hemodynamics and myocardial blood flow. *Basic Res Cardiol* 1984, 79(5):531-541.

[32] Reilly PM, MacGowan S, Miyachi M, Schiller HJ, Vickers S, Bulkley GB: Mesenteric vasoconstriction in cardiogenic shock in pigs. *Gastroenterology* 1992, 102(6):1968-1979.

[33] Kang H, Manasia A, Rajamani S, Rajaram SS, Hannon E, Lu Y, Oropello JM, Benjamin E: Intravenous iloprost increases mesenteric blood flow in experimental acute nonocclusive mesenteric ischemia. *Crit Care Med* 2002, 30(11):2528-2534.

[34] Aneman A, Treggiari MM, Burgener D, Laesser M, Strasser S, Hadengue A: Tezosentan normalizes hepatomesenteric perfusion in a porcine model of cardiac tamponade. *Acta Anaesthesiol Scand* 2009, 53(2):203-209.

[35] Burgener D, Laesser M, Treggiari-Venzi M, Oi Y, Jolliet P, Strasser S, Hadengue A, Aneman A: Endothelin-1 blockade corrects mesenteric

hypoperfusion in a porcine low cardiac output model. *Crit Care Med* 2001, 29(8):1615-1620.

[36] Snygg J, Aneman A, Pettersson A, Fandriks L: Jejunal mucosal nitric oxide production and substrate dependency during acute mesenteric hypoperfusion in pigs. *Crit Care Med* 2000, 28(7):2563-2566.

[37] Park M, Maciel AT, Noritomi DT, Brunialti MK, Salomao R, Schettino GP, Azevedo LC: Is persistent hypotension after transient cardiogenic shock associated with an inflammatory response? *Braz J Med Biol Res* 2008, 41(8):648-656.

[38] Vass A, Suveges G, Erces D, Nogrady M, Varga G, Foldesi I, Futakuchi M, Imai M, Okada N, Okada H et al: Inflammatory activation after experimental cardiac tamponade. *Eur Surg Res* 2013, 51(1-2):1-13.

[39] Erces D, Nogrady M, Nagy E, Varga G, Vass A, Suveges G, Imai M, Okada N, Okada H, Boros M et al: Complement C5A antagonist treatment improves the acute circulatory and inflammatory consequences of experimental cardiac tamponade. *Crit Care Med* 2013, 41(11):e344-351.

[40] Kuwagata Y, Oda J, Matsuyama S, Nishino M, Hashiguchi N, Ogura H, Tanaka H, Sugimoto H: Interleukin-1beta alters the oxygen delivery-oxygen consumption relationship in rabbits by increasing the slope of the supply-independent line. *Shock* 2000, 14(2):193-199.

[41] Viires N, Sillye G, Aubier M, Rassidakis A, Roussos C: Regional blood flow distribution in dog during induced hypotension and low cardiac output. Spontaneous breathing versus artificial ventilation. *J Clin Invest* 1983, 72(3):935-947.

In: Cardiac Tamponade
Editor: Cameron L. Pittman
ISBN: 978-1-63482-787-4

Chapter 4

Malignant Pericardial Effusion: Current Diagnosis and Treatment

Ranjit Kumar Chaudhary, MBBS[1], Smith Giri, MBBS[2], Ranjan Pathak, MD,[3] Sumit Dahal, MBBS,[4] and Vijaya Raj Bhatt, MBBS[5*]

[1]Department of Medicine, Institute of Medicine, Tribhuvan University, Kathmandu, Nepal
[2]Department of Medicine, University of Tennessee Health Science Center, Memphis, TN
[3]Department of Medicine, Reading Health System, Reading, PA
[4]Department of Internal Medicine, Interfaith Medical Center, NY, US
[5]Department of Internal Medicine, Division of Hematology and Oncology, University of Nebraska Medical Center, Omaha, NE

Abstract

Pericardium is a common site for neoplastic involvement that occurs due to direct local invasion by malignancy or metastatic spread via the

* Correspondence: Vijaya Raj Bhatt, University of Nebraska Medical Center. Department of Internal Medicine, Division of Hematology-Oncology. 987680 Nebraska Medical Center. Omaha, NE 68198-7680. Phone: (402) 559-5388. Fax: (402) 559-6520. Email: vijaya.bhatt@unmc.edu

lymphatics or bloodstream. Malignant involvement of the pericardium or occasionally treatment of malignancy can cause pericardial effusion. Pericardial effusion can be asymptomatic or cause chest discomfort, dyspnea, tachycardia, hypotension and cardiogenic shock, with increasing amount of fluid. Electrocardiogram, chest x-ray, echocardiography and cardiac catheterization can all aid in diagnosis of pericardial effusion but pericardial fluid and biopsy with histologic and cytologic analysis is required for diagnosis on underlying malignancy.

Prognosis for patients with malignant pericardial effusion is primarily dictated by the underlying disease. Since outcome is usually poor, goal of treatment is palliation of symptoms and prevention of recurrence of effusion. Pericardiocentesis is useful for prevention and treatment of cardiac tamponade but inadequate in itself because of a high rate of recurrence even when followed by extended tube drainage. Pericardial sclerosis has good success rate but high rate of complications such as arrhythmias and pericardial constriction. This makes it less preferred option than pericardial drainage; however, it may be useful for those, who are unfit for any surgical intervention. Cisplatin and tetracycline are most widely used sclerosing agents. Confirmed malignant pericardial effusion can be treated with relatively high doses of intrapericardial chemotherapy with minimal systemic side effects but the disease is restricted to only pericardium on a rare occasion. In disseminated malignancy, intrapericardial chemotherapy can improve symptoms of a hemodynamically significant effusion but other more effective and inexpensive treatment modalities may also be available.

Surgical treatment appears to result in better clinical outcome but selection of healthier patients may be confounding the results. Pericardial fenestration is the most commonly performed surgical procedure that employs subxiphoid, video-assisted thoracic surgery (VATS) and mini-thoracotomy approaches. This has an overall success rate of 93%, recurrence rate of 6% and perioperative complication rate of 4%. Subxiphoid approach can be performed under local anesthesia and does not require single-lung ventilation procedure unlike during VATS. Pericardiectomy is performed using VATS and is the second most commonly performed surgical procedure with almost 100% success rate but with a perioperative complication rate of up to 10%. Pericardio-peritoneal shunt as a treatment of malignant pericardial effusion has been reported as a safe and effective treatment but the small study population mandates further confirmatory studies. Percutaneous balloon pericardiotomy has good outcome, can be performed under local anesthesia and allows early discharge. It is useful in poor surgical candidates but has higher complications (up to 32%), which include a risk of pleural effusion, fever and pneumothorax. Outcomes tend to be better in the high-volume centers.

In conclusion, there is a paucity of high-quality studies and a lack of therapeutic options with significant impact on survival of patients with malignant pericardial effusion. Safe, cost effective and durable palliative treatment as well as treatment strategies that can prolong survival meaningfully are needed.

Keywords: Malignant pericardial effusion, pericardiocentesis, pericardiectomy, pericardial window, intrapericardial chemotherapy, cytology, pericardial sclerosis, percutaneous balloon pericardiectomy, pericardial-peritoneal shunt, video-assisted thoracoscopic surgery

Introduction

Neoplastic involvement of pericardium and pericardial effusion are common causes of morbidity in cancer patients. Lung cancer, breast cancer and lymphoma are among the most common malignancies associated with pericardial effusion. Treatment of malignant pericardial effusion is difficult due to its tendency to recur despite therapy. Prognosis for patients with malignant pericardial effusion is primarily dictated by the underlying malignancy but is usually poor. Hence, the goal of treatment is palliation of symptoms and prevention of recurrence of effusion [1]. In this chapter, we discuss the epidemiology, clinical presentation, diagnostic and therapeutic approaches of malignant pericardial effusion.

Epidemiology

Involvement of pericardium by malignancy is observed in 2%-4% of the general population and 7%-21% of cancer patients; however, the incidence of clinically significant effusion is much lower [1, 2]. Symptomatic pericardial effusion with unknown diagnosis after routine investigation can be initial manifestation of malignancy in nearly 20% of cases but cardiac tamponade as an initial symptom of malignancy is rare. Only 12%–25% of patients with neoplastic involvement of pericardium have pericardial effusion, of which only a few patients develop cardiac tamponade. Primary neoplasms of pericardium are extremely rare and include malignant mesotheliomas, fibrosarcomas, lymphangiomas and hemangiomas [3]. More than 80% of malignancies involving pericardium include metastasis or local spread from lung cancer, breast cancer, lymphoma (Hodgkin's and Non-Hodgkin's) and leukemia (table 1). However, it is important to understand that approximately 50% of all pericardial diseases in cancer patients is secondary to nonmalignant etiologies such as radiation or drugs used to treat cancer [4].

Table 1. Primary site of malignancy causing pericardial effusion

Malignancy	Percent of cases of malignant pericardial effusion	
	Press et al. [5]	Wiles et al. [6]
Lung	36.5 %	30%
Breast	22.3%	23%
Leukemia and lymphoma	17.2%	27%
Sarcomas	3.5%	3%
Melanoma	2.7%	2.4%
Stomach	2.0%	2.4%
Carcinoma of unknown origin	2.0%	3%
Renal	1.9%	1.6%
Others	11.7%	7.6%

Pathogenesis

Pericardium is a tough double-layered membrane covering the heart; the two layers enclose a potential space called pericardial cavity that contains tiny amount of fluid, usually less than 50 ml, to prevent friction between the two layers. Pericardial effusion occurs due to accumulation of fluid in the pericardial cavity; an inability to compensate for the increased amount of fluid can lead to hemodynamic compromise [7].

Pericardial effusion in malignancy can occur due to involvement of the pericardium either by direct extension of tumor such as from lung and esophagus or hematogenous or lymphatic dissemination of distant tumor.[8]Tumor cells infiltrating pericardium can cause irritation of pericardial membranes, which promote fluid secretion leading to pericardial effusion. Tumor can also obstruct venous drainage leading to an increase in the hydrostatic pressure and decrease in the reabsorption of interstitial fluid, thus resulting in pericardial effusion [7].

Pressure effect of tumor on lymphatic vessels can also cause pericardial effusion. Hematological malignancy can spread to the pericardium by a hematogenous route while malignancies that seed to mediastinal lymph node can spread via lymphatics.

Rarely, hemorrhagic effusion can occur as a result of intrapericardial extramedullary hematopoiesis in chronic myelomonocytic leukemia or the advanced stages of chronic myelogenous leukemia. Adverse effects of radiotherapy or chemotherapeutic agents (e.g. busulfan, cyclophosphamide or imatinib) can also result in pericardial effusion. Immunosuppression from malignancy or its treatment can predispose patients to opportunistic infections, which can also cause pericardial effusion. Lastly, hypoalbuminemia associated with malignancy can lead to effusion as a result of decreased osmotic pressure. [8]

Clinical Manifestation

Pericardial effusion can often be asymptomatic or present with non-specific symptoms such as fatigue, chest discomfort and dyspnea. Increasing amount of fluid in pericardial space can result in cardiac tamponade and may present as hypotension and cardiogenic shock [8]. Malignant infiltration of pericardium can result in rapid hemorrhagic effusion and cardiac tamponade, whereas inflammation of pericardium secondary to radiotherapy or chemotherapy frequently causes a slower accumulation of fluid [4]. Hence, malignant involvement of pericardium should always be thought as a possible cause of rapidly increasing or recurrent pericardial effusion that do not respond to non-steroidal anti-inflammatory drugs [8].

Physical examination findings of advanced pericardial effusion and tamponade include jugular venous distension, pulsus paradoxus (decrease in systolic arterial pressure more than 10 mmHg on inspiration), pulsus alternans and muffled heart sounds but these are not specific for malignant pericardial effusion [4]. Patients may also present with signs and symptoms of the underlying malignancy.

Diagnosis

Although clinical examination can give a clue to diagnose pericardial effusion, imaging tests are important in confirming the diagnosis. Chest x-ray is a simple diagnostic test but has limited usefulness due to its poor sensitivity and specificity. Chest x-ray may show an enlarged cardiac silhouette with clear lung field, mediastinal widening, hilar mass or pericardial fat pad displacement. Pleural effusion may be seen in 50% of patients with malignant pericardial effusion [2, 4].

Electrocardiogram (EKG), although abnormal in many cases, demonstrates nonspecific changes. EKG findings include sinus tachycardia, nonspecific ST-T wave changes, PR depression and premature ventricular contraction. Less common but more specific findings include low-voltage tracing (amplitude <0.5 mV in limb leads) and electrical alterations (beat to beat variation in amplitude of QRS complex and P wave) [4].

Echocardiography is frequently used for initial evaluation of cardiac function and pericardial effusion. It is non-invasive and highly sensitive in diagnosing pericardial effusion and assessing hemodynamic compromise. Echocardiography may show right atrial and ventricular collapse, decrease in left ventricular size and inspiratory increase in right-sided pressures. Echocardiographic finding of right atrial collapse has a sensitivity of up to 60% and a specificity of up to 68%, whereas ventricular collapse has a sensitivity of up to 48% and a specificity of 84-100% for the diagnosis of cardiac tamponade [2, 4].

Computed tomography (CT) of chest offers additional advantages in diagnosis of pericardial effusion, which include higher sensitivity to detect small pericardial effusion (as less as 50 ml of fluid), ability to provide information on anatomic structure of pericardium and surrounding structure such as vessels, lymph nodes, lung parenchyma and mediastinal pleura. Pericardial thickening and mediastinal lymphadenopathy along with pericardial effusion are often suggestive of malignant pericardial effusion. Contrast-enhanced helical CT of chest and magnetic resonance imaging (MRI) are particularly useful when pericardial thickening or loculated or hemorrhagic effusion is suspected. MRI of chest has good resolution and can be more informative than the CT of chest or echocardiography. [9, 10] MRI images can be improved by altering tissue signals by using pulse sequence, which is a set of computer instructions and algorithms that prepare and generate a magnetic resonance signal. Most commonly used pulse sequences for cardiac imaging are spin-echo and gradient-recalled echo cine images [11]. The appearance of hemorrhagic and non-hemorrhagic pericardial fluid is different on spin-echo images and gradient-recalled echo cine images. Nonhemorrhagic fluid has low signal intensity, whereas hemorraghic fluid has high intensity on T1-weighted spin-echo images. These findings are reversed in gradient-recalled echo cine images: nonhemorrhagic fluid has high intensity and hemorrhagic fluid has low intensity [3].

Right heart catheterization is useful for evaluation of the effects of pericardial effusion on cardiac function. Although not routinely performed, it is also a definitive test for diagnosis of cardiac tamponade. Increased right atrial pressure and equalization of diastolic pressures in all cardiac chambers, noted during right heart catheterization, is confirmatory of cardiac tamponade [4].

Increased accumulation of radioactive compound (^{67}Ga-citrate, ^{99m}Tm-pertechnate) in pericardial cavity may suggest a diagnosis of malignant pericardial effusion in patients with metastatic disease. Occasionally, however, benign pericardial effusion can also have these findings and mimic malignant pericardial effusion. In current clinical practice, a nuclear scan is of limited value due to the availability of better tests for evaluation of pericardial effusion [12, 13].

Once pericardial effusion is confirmed, pericardial fluid should be analyzed to diagnose the underlying etiology. In malignant pericardial effusion, accumulated fluid can be serous, serosanguinous or hemorrhagic. Fluid chemistry analysis and microbiologic evaluation including bacterial, viral and fungal cultures can aid in diagnosis. Although bloody pericardial effusion with specific gravity >1.016 and protein level >3g/dL is highly suggestive of malignant effusion, histologic and cytologic demonstration of tumor cells in pericardial fluid and biopsy are needed for definitive diagnosis of malignant pericardial effusion [4]. However, cytology can be falsely negative, and malignant lymphocytes may be indistinguishable from reactive lymphocytes seen in inflammatory pericardial effusion [1]. Cytology has a sensitivity that varies from 54% to 90% [14]. The diagnostic yield of cytology depends on accurate sampling and cytopreparatory techniques. Also addition of ancillary studies (immunocytochemistry, flow cytometry, morphometry and cytogenetics) can be helpful in establishing etiology of pericardial effusion, particularly in patients with hematological malignancies [1].

Tumor markers can be a useful tool in establishing etiology, especially when cytology of pericardial fluid is negative or diagnosis is equivocal. Carcinoembryonic antigen (CEA), serum cytokeratin 19 fragments (CYFRA

21-1), neuron-specific enolase (NSE), CA 125, CA 15-3 and CA 19-9 tumor markers in the effusion can aid in diagnosis of pericardial effusion due to solid tumors. However, the cut-off values of these tumor markers are not well defined and sensitivity and specificity of these tumor markers are variable. Combination of two or more tumor markers can increase the diagnostic value [1]. The optimal cut-off value used for CYFRA 21-1is >100ng/ml and has a sensitivity and specificity of 74% and 92%, whereas optimal cut-off value used for CEA is >5ng/ml with sensitivity and specificity of 72% and 97%. Combining pericardial fluid cytology to CEA level measurement (cut-off >5ng/ml) increases sensitivity to 92% and specificity to 94%, while combining pericardial fluid cytology to CYFRA 21-1 level measurement (cut-off >100ng/ml) increases sensitivity to 95% and specificity to 92%. Combining pericardial fluid cytology and tumor markers such as CEA and CYFRA 21-1 to evaluate malignant pericardial effusion increases the accuracy of the test to >90% [15].

Pericardioscopy allows access to the parts of the pericardial cavity that is not possible through the subxiphoid window. It has a sensitivity of 97%, which can increase the probability of diagnosis of malignant pericardial effusion. In a study of 44 patients with malignant pericardial effusion, nearly 22% of patients had a non-diagnostic pericardial fluid cytology and pericardial window biopsy; in these patients, pericardioscopy helped to clinch a diagnosis by allowing better visualization and guiding pericardial biopsy. However, the procedure has a perioperative mortality rate of 3.5% and a postoperative morbidity rate of 6%. Therefore, the procedure is contraindicated in unfit patients or patients with significant comorbidities [16, 17].

Vascular endothelial growth factor (VEGF) levels are markedly elevated in malignant versus benign pericardial effusion. VEGF level in pericardial fluid, thus, can help in differentiating malignant from benign pericardial effusions [18]. Limited studies are available regarding the usefulness of osteoprotegerin and TNF-related apoptosis-inducing ligand levels for diagnosis of malignant pericardial effusion [19].

Prognosis

Prognosis for patients with malignant pericardial effusion is usually poor and primarily depends upon the underlying stage of malignancy, tissue diagnosis and response to treatment [20]. The median survival time is significantly shorter in patients with an abnormal results of pericardial fluid cytology than in those patients with a normal cytology [21, 22]. High serum calcium and a low albumin/globulin ratio is also associated with a poorer prognosis [23].

Treatment

Although short term risk of death from effusion can be prevented by timely management of malignant pericardial effusion, overall quality of life and survival with currently available therapeutic options is usually poor. The goal of treatment is palliation of symptoms and prevention of recurrence of effusion. The status of the underlying malignancy and patient's overall health determine the overall survival and should also guide the choice of treatment modality for the malignant pericardial effusion (Table 2; Figure 1) [24].

Pericardiocentesis

Echocardiogram-guided pericardiocentesis is very safe and efficacious as an initial treatment modality but is associated with a high risk of recurrence. The procedure is also difficult in obese patients and patients with loculated posterior effusion or minimal effusion [25]. Initial pericardiocentesis of malignant pericardial effusion results in success in nearly two-third of cases but recurrence of effusion can be as high as 50%. [24]. Pericardiocentesis followed by extended catheter drainage has a resolution rate of up to 55% while remaining cases need further intervention for treatment of recurrence. Complications can occur in nearly 12% of cases; arrhythmias are the most common complication [26]. Prolonged drainage is usually done for 4-5 days; catheter should not be removed until drainage is less than 20-30ml in 24 hour [8, 27].

Pericardial Sclerosis

Pericardial sclerosis has a good success rate but also has a higher rate of complications including constrictive pericarditis. Therefore, it is a less preferred option than pericardial drainage; however, it may be useful for patients, who are unfit for any surgical intervention. Cisplatin, tetracycline, thiotepa, bleomycin, mitomycin C and mitoxantrone are frequently used agents. Tetracycline and doxycycline are pure sclerosing agents, which probably induce irritation, inflammation and subsequent fibrosis [1]. Additionally, cytostatic activity of tetracycline has been suggested to contribute to its therapeutic effect [28].

These agents can cause severe chest pain, which may require opioid analgesics to control pain. Bleomycin and thiotepa have both antineoplastic and sclerosing effects and have good success rates with fewer side effects [1]. Treatment of malignant pericardial effusion with relatively high doses of intrapericardial chemotherapy has only minimal systemic side effects but the disease is rarely restricted to pericardium alone. Etoposide, 5-fluorouracil, cisplatin, mitomycin C and mitoxantrone are frequently utilized local chemotherapeutic agents. In disseminated malignancy, intrapericardial chemotherapy can improve the symptoms of effusion but other treatment modalities available may be more effective and inexpensive. Cisplatin is the most widely used agent with a success rate of nearly 90% with a relatively low rate of effusion recurrence (9%) and relatively modest procedure-related morbidity (14%). The intrapericardial instillation of tetracycline and cisplatin has similar overall success rate (88% vs. 90%) and the risk of recurrence (9% for both) but the adverse events occur more frequently with tetracycline (45% vs. 14%). Thiotepa has a success rate of 91% but slightly lower complication rate of 7%. Bleomycin and mitoxantrone have largely similar success rates as cisplatin but have higher rates of complications. Mitomycin C is less frequently used due to a lower success rate and higher complication rate [26].

Intrapericardial instillation of radioactive agent (^{32}P-colloid) for treatment of malignant pericardial effusion has good response rate with minimal complications. In a prospective study, patients (n=36), who developed pericardial effusion after receiving chemotherapy with or without radiotherapy, were treated with intrapericardial ^{32}P-colloid instillation. This resulted in a complete remission rate of 94% for a median period of 8 months (3-24 months) with no early complication. All patients, who were in complete remission, died of cancer progression but had no signs of pericardial effusion at the time of death. The two patients who did not respond had rapid formation of pericardial effusion and died shortly after ^{32}P-colloid instillation [29]. Intrapericardial instillation of radioactive chromic phosphate has also been used in the past with a success rate of 71% [30]. Intrapericardial instillation of cytokines (interferon-α2b, interferon-β and interleukin-2) for the management of malignant pericardial effusion has also been reported [8].

Table 2. Comparison of different treatment modalities for pericardial effusion

Treatment modality	Number of patients	Age in years, median (range)	Outcome	Complication
[24]Pericardiocentesis [a]	100	47 (17-82)	41% recurrence at 1-year.	Catheter occlusion (5%) and vagal hypotension (3%).
[49]Intrapericardial cisplatin injection [b]	42	58	17% recurrence at 6 months.	Myocardial ischemia in 2.4%
[50]Pericardial window, VATS approach [c]	62	58 (19-79)	11% recurrence rate.	Post-operative ventilation support (2%)
[51]Pericardial window, subxiphoid approach [d]	155	-	No recurrence at 107 days	None reported
[36]Mediastinoscope-controlled parasternal fenestration [e]	22	57 (26-72)	No recurrence at 2 months[f]	Postoperative mortality (4.5%), transient arrhythmias (14%) and transient accumulation of pericardial fluid (4.5%)
[38]Pericardiectomy [g]	11	62	No recurrence at 13 months	-
[39]Pericardio-peritoneal shunt [h]	4	57	No recurrence at 3 months	No immediate or long–term complication.
[32]Percutaneous balloon pericardiotomy [i]	50	58	4% recurrence at 3 months	Fever (12%), new pleural effusion (4%), pneumothorax (4%), right ventricular tear (2%) and conversion to surgery (4%).
[44]OK-432 intrapericardial instillation [j]	10	60 (34-68)	100% resolution rate with no recurrence at 329 days	Fever (60%), chest pain (50%) and arrhythmias (30%)
[29]Intrapericardial ^{32}P-colloid [k]	36	62 (42-86)	94% resolution rate; duration of response of 8 months	Transient tachycardia in 3%

Mediastinoscope-controlled parasternal fenestration, pericardiectomy and pericarido-peritoneal shunt resulted in a resolution rate of 100%, whereas percutaneous balloon pericardiotomy resulted in a resolution rate of 92%.

[a]Intrapericardial instillation of interferon alpha- 2b in 24% but no significant difference in resolution rate between group receiving interferon alpha-2b and group not receiving it.

[b]Single intrapericardial instillation at dose 30mg/m^2 for 24 hrs. followed by evacuation.

[c]Survival was significantly lower in those with positive pericardial fluid cytology.

[d]27% of cases had malignant pericardial tamponade

[e]Malignant origin of pericardial effusion could not be verified in 14%.

[f]Survival status available in 64%.

[g]Mean total resected area of 16.4 cm^2. Resection performed using VATS. Local chemotherapy was given in 45% of cases

[h]Average hospital stay was significantly lower compared to subxiphoid or anterior thoracotomy pericardial window

[i]Cardiac tamponade in 72% and large effusion in 28%. 88% had history of malignancy.

[j]70% required 5KE (Klinische Einheit) unit while 30% required repeat instillation, thus receiving a total of 10 KE unit of OK-432.

[k]Effusion completely removed prior to instillation of ^{32}P-colloid. Single dose of 5mCi was successful in 58% while 39% required repeat dose of 5mCi after 2 weeks.

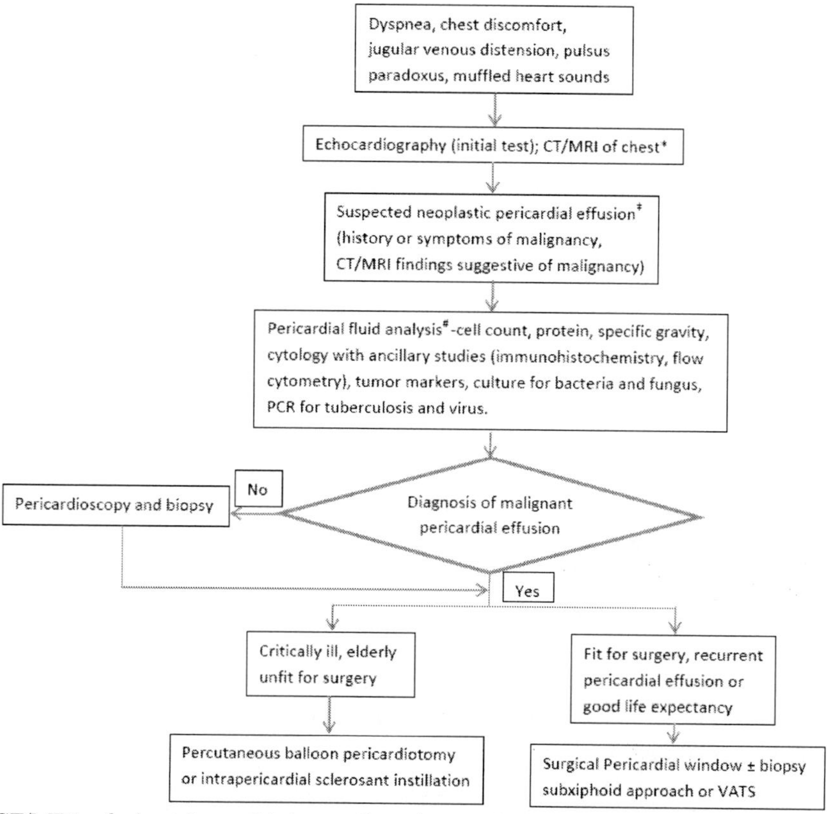

*CT/MRI of chest is useful in small and posteriorly located loculated pericardial effusion. CT/MRI provides information about pericardium and surrounding structure that may help to establish etiology.

‡ Urgent pericardiocentesis may be needed for patients with cardiac tamponade and large malignant pericardial effusion.

Specific gravity >1.015, protein level >3 g/dL, fluid/serum protein ratio >0.5, LDH >200 mg/dL, fluid/serum LDH ratio >0.6 are suggestive of exudate. Although these parameters are validated for pleural fluid; these have been commonly used for pericardial fluid as well. [48] Hemorrhagic fluid with specific gravity >1.016 and protein level >3 mg/dL is highly suggestive of malignant effusion.[4] Tumor markers CEA >5 ng/mL or CYFRA 21-1>100 ng/mL have good sensitivity and specificity [15].

Figure 1. Management Algorithm for suspected malignant pericardial effusion [1, 3, 4, 9, 15, 26, 32, 46-48].

Surgical Interventions

Surgical treatment appears to result in better clinical outcomes in select patients but selection of healthier patients as surgical candidates may be confounding the results. Underlying malignancy (lung cancer has worst outcome), presence of a pleural effusion and positive pathologic or cytologic findings are preoperative factors associated with lower survival in patients undergoing surgical management of malignant pericardial effusion [31]. Three different surgical approaches used for treatment of malignant pericardial effusion include pericardial fenestration, pericardiectomy and pericardio-peritoneal shunt insertion. Pericardial fenestration surgery, the most commonly performed surgery, creates a window in pericardium that allows drainage of pericardial fluid into pleural space. Pericardial fenestration is commonly performed using three different approaches- subxiphoid, video-assisted thoracic surgery (VATS) and mini-thoracotomy [26]. Transthoracic windowing procedure or total pericardiectomy does not offer significant advantage over subxiphoid pericardial windowing but increases postoperative morbidity (67% vs. 10%) [32]. Therefore, this is no longer a preferred approach. Pericardial fenestration surgery has an overall success rate of 93%, recurrence rate of 6% and perioperative complication rate of 4%. Subxiphoid approach is the most commonly used technique and can be performed under local anesthesia. VATS is performed under general anesthesia and requires single-lung ventilation procedure and a thoracoscope inserted into thorax to guide excision of a portion of pericardium to create a pericardial window. VATS may be difficult to perform in critically ill patients. Subxiphoid approach, VATS and left mini-thoracotomy have comparable success rate (93% vs. 91% vs. 96%, respectively), recurrence rate (5% vs. 9% vs. 4%, respectively) and complication rate (4% vs. 5% vs. 11%, respectively) [26]. Subxiphoid approach, compared to left mini-thoracotomy approach, requires shorter operative time and length of hospital stay and additionally, has lower risk of infection and postoperative pain [33]. Due to lower chances of recurrence with left mini-thoracotomy, it may be preferred over subxiphoid and VATS approach in patients with a high probability of long-term survival [34]. Patients with symptomatic pericardial effusions, who are treated with open subxiphoid pericardial drainage, have lower risk of recurrence (5% vs. 16%, p =0.002) and lower hospital-related mortality (11% vs. 23%, p=0.01) compared to patients treated with percutaneous catheter drainage [35]. In a small study (n=22), mediastinoscope-controlled parasternal fenestration showed success rate of 100% with transient dysrhythmias in 14% of patients. However, one patient died during postoperative period. The small size of study warrants further investigations to establish its value [36]. Permanent placement of port-system after thoracoscopically creating a pericardial window has been tried for recurrent malignant pericardial effusion in patients with advanced malignancy but high procedural mortality of 7.5% makes it a less preferred option [37].

Pericardiectomy is usually performed using VATS, and it is the second most commonly performed surgical procedure with almost 100% success rate but with a perioperative complication rate of up to 10%. Good visualization during VATS approach increases the certainty of the procedure and can decrease the length of hospital stay; it is also less painful compared to other surgical procedures [26, 38].

Pericardio-peritoneal shunt is a tube like structure with an inflow end and an outflow end; both ends are connected to a pumping chamber in the center. Pericardio-peritoneal shunt placement is performed under local anesthesia and uses a vertical incision over xiphoid process. The inflow end of shunt is placed in pericardial space, a subcutaneous pocket is created for the pumping chamber and outflow end of shunt is tunneled subcutaneously into peritoneal cavity. Pericardio-peritoneal shunt as a treatment of malignant pericardial effusion has been reported as a safe and effective treatment in a few cases but mandates confirmatory studies [39, 40].

Pericardio-peritoneal window has been used for treatment of recurrent benign and malignant pericardial effusions. An opening is created using subxiphoid approach in pericardium and peritoneum in area covering dome of liver, and the two linings are sutured together to allow drainage of pericardial fluid. The dome of diaphragm prevents herniation of abdominal contents into pericardial space. Effectiveness of this therapeutic option has only been demonstrated in small studies and needs further investigation to establish its usefulness [41, 42].

Percutaneous balloon pericardiotomy is a method of creating a pericardial window by inflating a balloon catheter passed over a guide wire into pericardial space. This allows drainage of pericardial fluid into pleural space. This treatment modality has good effusion resolution rate (90%), is less invasive and can be performed under local anesthesia. It is useful in poor surgical candidates but has higher complications (up to 32%), which include a risk of pleural effusion (16%), fever (12%) and pneumothorax (4%). Outcomes tend to be better in the high-volume centers [26, 32].

Radiotherapy

External beam radiation at doses 200 to 4,000 rad can be used as a therapeutic option for malignant pericardial effusion and is particularly useful for effusions secondary to radiosensitive tumors such as leukemias and lymphomas. Improvement is seen in up to two-third of patients but higher doses of radiation can cause pancarditis. The time required for response and duration of therapy makes it a less preferred option [4, 43].

Experimental Approaches

A number of experimental modalities have emerged in recent years. The most promising therapies include the use of OK-432 and intrapericardial immunotherapy. OK-432 is penicillin- and heat-treated lyophilized powder of the substrain of *Streptococcus pyogenes* A3. It can stimulate cell-mediated immunity to result in a direct cytotoxic effect on malignant cells. There are limited studies showing usefulness of intrapericardial instillation of OK-432 in treatment of malignant pericardial effusion. In a study (n=10), only 30% of the patients required retreatment with OK-432 due to reaccumulation of fluid; such approach resulted in resolution of effusion. Fever and chest pain were common adverse effects, which occurred in more than one-half of the patients but were controlled with antipyretics alone. Twenty percent experienced hypotension that was successfully controlled with vasopressor drugs. Arrhythmias occurred in 30% of patients but were not life-threatening. Although 70% of patients had thickened pericardium, none of the patients developed constrictive pericarditis [44].

Intrapericardial immunotherapy using autologous lymphocytes directed against infiltrating tumor is a novel therapy. The tumor infiltrating lymphocytes is obtained from pericardial fluid and cultured in vitro. These lymphocytes are expanded using interleukin-2 and are infused into pericardial space every 2 weeks after an initial pericardiocentesis. In a study (n=6), it resulted in regression of pericardial effusion in all four patients, who received immunotherapy. Conversely, pericardial effusion reaccumulated in two cases, who did not receive the novel therapy due to inadequate culture growth and poor performance status. Grade 1 fever was the most common side effect [45]. Given the small sample, more studies are needed to establish the role of tumor-infiltrating lymphocyte infusion in management of pericardial effusion.

Combined surgical and medical approach for malignant pericardial effusion is not well studied. However, small studies failed to show improvement in therapeutic response or survival in patients with malignant pericardial effusion who received intrapericardial injections of sclerosant (mitomycin C, tetracycline or doxorubicin) in addition to creation of subxiphoid pericardial window [1].

Conclusion

Pericardium is occasionally involved in malignancy and can cause significant morbidity in cancer patients. Malignant pericardial effusion can be asymptomatic or have non-specific symptoms. Since patients with a history of malignancy can have pericardial effusion due to non-malignant cause, establishing the etiology of pericardial effusion is important but can be difficult. Although various clinical and imaging diagnostic modalities are available, pericardial fluid cytology and pericardial biopsy are particularly valuable in establishing etiology.

Since treatment of malignant pericardial effusion may not influence long term survival, the goal of treatment is to control symptoms. Due to high rate of effusion recurrence after pericardiocentesis, other more definitive measures are needed. Surgical methods are preferred in patients with malignant pericardial effusion due to lower chances of recurrence. However, surgical options may not be feasible for patients, who are critically ill or elderly patients unable to tolerate surgery. Pericardial instillation of sclerosant and chemotherapeutic drug or percutaneous balloon pericardiotomy can be helpful treatment options in such patients. Novel therapeutic measures such as intrapericardial immunotherapy with OK-432 and autologous lymphocytes directed against infiltrating tumor cells require further studies to establish their role.

There are limited diagnostic and therapeutic options for safe and durable palliative management of malignant pericardial effusion. Treatment strategies that can prolong survival meaningfully are needed.

Conflict of Interest/Funding: None

References

[1] Lestuzzi C. Neoplastic pericardial disease: old and current strategies for diagnosis and management. *World journal of cardiology* 2010;2:270.

[2] Shepherd FA. Malignant pericardial effusion. *Current opinion in oncology* 1997;9:170-4.

[3] Refaat MM, Katz WE. Neoplastic pericardial effusion. *Clinical cardiology* 2011;34:593-8.

[4] Retter A. Pericardial disease in the oncology patient. *Heart disease* (Hagerstown, Md) 2001;4:387-91.

[5] Press OW, Livingston R. Management of malignant pericardial effusion and tamponade. *JAMA* 1987;257:1088-92.

[6] Wilkes JD, Fidias P, Vaickus L, Perez RP. Malignancy-related pericardial effusion. 127 cases from the roswell park cancer institute. *Cancer* 1995;76:1377-87.

[7] Mangan C. Malignant pericardial effusions: pathophysiology and clinical correlates. *Oncology nursing forum*; 1992. p. 1215-21.

[8] Burazor I, Imazio M, Markel G, Adler Y. Malignant pericardial effusion. *Cardiology* 2013;124:224-32.

[9] Sun JS, Park KJ, Kang DK. CT findings in patients with pericardial effusion: differentiation of malignant and benign disease. *American Journal of Roentgenology* 2010;194:W489-W94.

[10] Chiles C, Woodard PK, Gutierrez FR, Link KM. Metastatic Involvement of the Heart and Pericardium: CT and MR Imaging 1. *Radiographics* 2001;21:439-49.

[11] Musani MH, Chaudhry A, Voros S, Poon M. The Role of Cardiac Magnetic Resonance Imaging in Cardiology Consultation. *Evidence-Based Cardiology* Consult: Springer; 2014:221-37.

[12] Simpson AJ. Malignant Pericardial Effusion Diagnosed by Combined 67Ga-Citrate and 99mTc-Pertechnetate Scintigraphy. Clinical nuclear medicine 1978;3:445-6.

[13] Valdez VA, Jacobstein JG. Visualization of a malignant pericardial effusion with Tc-99m-EHDP. *Clinical nuclear medicine* 1980;5:210-2.

[14] Ben-Horin S, Bank I, Guetta V, Livneh A. Large symptomatic pericardial effusion as the presentation of unrecognized cancer: a study in 173 consecutive patients undergoing pericardiocentesis. *Medicine* 2006;85:49-53.

[15] Szturmowicz M, Tomkowski W, Fijalkowska A, et al. Diagnostic utility of CYFRA 21-1 and CEA assays in pericardial fluid for the recognition of neoplastic pericarditis. *The International journal of biological markers* 2004;20:43-9.

[16] Porte HL, Janecki-Delebecq TJ, Finzi L, Métois DG, Millaire A, Wurtz AJ. Pericardoscopy for primary management of pericardial effusion in cancer patients. *European journal of cardio-thoracic surgery* 1999;16:287-91.

[17] Millaire A, Wurtz A, de Groote P, Saudemont A, Chambon A, Ducloux G. Malignant pericardial effusions: usefulness of pericardioscopy. *American heart journal* 1992;124:1030-4.

[18] Karatolios K, Pankuweit S, Moosdorf RG, Maisch B. Vascular endothelial growth factor in malignant and benign pericardial effusion. *Clinical cardiology* 2012;35:377-81.

[19] Karatolios K, Pankuweit S, Goettsch C, et al. Osteoprotegerin (OPG) and TNF-related apoptosis-inducing ligand (TRAIL) levels in malignant and benign pericardial effusions. *Clinical biochemistry* 2012;45:237-42.

[20] Dequanter D, Lothaire P, Berghmans T, Sculier J-P. Severe pericardial effusion in patients with concurrent malignancy: a retrospective analysis of prognostic factors influencing survival. *Annals of surgical oncology* 2008;15:3268-71.

[21] Jeong T-D, Jang S, Park C-J, Chi H-S. Prognostic relevance of pericardial effusion in patients with malignant diseases. The Korean journal of hematology 2012;47:237.

[22] Gornik HL, Gerhard-Herman M, Beckman JA. Abnormal cytology predicts poor prognosis in cancer patients with pericardial effusion. *Journal of clinical oncology* 2005;23:5211-6.

[23] Wang H-J, Hsu K-L, Chiang F-T, Tseng C-D, Tseng Y-Z, Liau C-S. Technical and prognostic outcomes of double-balloon pericardiotomy for large malignancy-related pericardial effusions. *CHEST Journal* 2002;122:893-9.

[24] Apodaca-Cruz Á, Villarreal-Garza C, Torres-Ávila B, et al. Effectiveness and prognosis of initial pericardiocentesis in the primary management of malignant pericardial effusion. *Interactive cardiovascular and thoracic surgery* 2010;11:154-61.

[25] Marcy P, Bondiau P, Brunner P. Percutaneous treatment in patients presenting with malignant cardiac tamponade. *European radiology* 2005;15:2000-9.

[26] Jama GM, Scarci M, Bowden J, Marciniak SJ. Palliative treatment for symptomatic malignant pericardial effusion. *Interactive cardiovascular and thoracic surgery* 2014:ivu267.

[27] Marshall MB. Symptomatic Malignant Pericardial Effusion: Surgical or Percutaneous Drainage? *Difficult Decisions in Thoracic Surgery*: Springer; 2011:453-9.

[28] Sauter C. Cytostatic activity of oxidized tetracycline in vitro: relevance for the treatment of malignant effusions? *British journal of cancer* 1988;57:514.

[29] Dempke W, Firusian N. Treatment of malignant pericardial effusion with 32P-colloid. British journal of cancer 1999;80:1955.

[30] Martini N, Freiman AH, Watson RC, Hilaris BS. Intrapericardial installation of radioactive chromic phosphate in malignant effusion. *American Journal of Roentgenology* 1977;128:639-41.

[31] Cullinane CA, Paz IB, Smith D, Carter N, Grannis FW. Prognostic factors in the surgical management of pericardial effusion in the patient with concurrent malignancy. *CHEST Journal* 2004;125:1328-34.

[32] Ziskind AA, Pearce AC, Lemmon CC, et al. Percutaneous balloon pericardiotomy for the treatment of cardiac tamponade and large pericardial effusions: description of technique and report of the first 50 cases. *Journal of the American College of Cardiology* 1993;21:1-5.

[33] Ibrahim Kasb M, Osama Rashwan M, Biomy R. Management of Malignant Pericardial Effusion: A comparative study of Subxiphoid versus Mini-thoracotomy Approach. EDITORIAL BOARD;21:49.

[34] Çelik S, Lestuzzi C, Cervesato E, et al. Systemic chemotherapy in combination with pericardial window has better outcomes in malignant pericardial effusions. *The Journal of thoracic and cardiovascular surgery* 2014.

[35] McDonald JM, Meyers BF, Guthrie TJ, Battafarano RJ, Cooper JD, Patterson GA. Comparison of open subxiphoid pericardial drainage with percutaneous catheter drainage for symptomatic pericardial effusion. *The Annals of thoracic surgery* 2003;76:811-6.

[36] Toth I, Szucs G, Molnar TF. Mediastinoscope-controlled parasternal fenestration of the pericardium: definitive surgical palliation of malignant pericardial effusion. *J Cardiothorac Surg* 2012;7:56.

[37] Melfi FM, Menconi GF, Chella A, Angeletti CA. The management of malignant pericardial effusions using permanently implanted devices. *European Journal of Cardio-Thoracic Surgery* 2002;21:345-7.

[38] Uramoto H, Hanagiri T. Video-assisted thoracoscopic pericardiectomy for malignant pericardial effusion. *Anticancer research* 2010;30:4691-4.

[39] Wang N, Feikes JR, Mogensen T, Vyhmeister EE, Bailey LL. Pericardioperitoneal shunt: an alternative treatment for malignant pericardial effusion. *The Annals of thoracic surgery* 1994;57:289-92.

[40] Marcy P, Magné N. Imaging of percutaneous pericardioperitoneal shunt in patient with malignant cardiac tamponade. JBR-BTR 2004;87:186-9.

[41] Kallianpur AA, Samra SS, Nimbran V, et al. Pericardial-peritoneal window: A novel palliative treatment for malignant and recurrent cardiac tamponade. *Indian journal of palliative care* 2013;19:116.

[42] Olson JE, Ryan MB, Blumenstock DA. Eleven years' experience with pericardial-peritoneal window in the management of malignant and benign pericardial effusions. *Annals of surgical oncology* 1995;2:165-9.

[43] Fairlamb D. External radiotherapy in the management of malignant pericardial effusion. *Clinical radiology* 1989;40:307-8.

[44] Imamura T, Tamura K, Takenaga M, Nagatomo Y, Ishikawa T, Nakagawa S. Intrapericardial ok-432 instillation for the management of malignant pericardial effusion. *Cancer* 1991;68:259-63.

[45] Toh U, Fujii T, Seki N, Niiya F, Shirouzu K, Yamana H. Characterization of IL-2-activated TILs and their use in intrapericardial immunotherapy in malignant pericardial effusion. *Cancer Immunology, Immunotherapy* 2006;55:1219-27.

[46] Maisch B, Rupp H, Ristic A, Pankuweit S. Pericardioscopy and epi-and pericardial biopsy—a new window to the heart improving etiological diagnoses and permitting targeted intrapericardial therapy. *Heart failure reviews* 2013;18:317-28.

[47] Swanson N, Mirza I, Wijesinghe N, Devlin G. Primary percutaneous balloon pericardiotomy for malignant pericardial effusion. *Catheterization and Cardiovascular Interventions* 2008;71:504-7.

[48] Imazio M, Adler Y. Management of pericardial effusion. *European heart journal* 2012:ehs372.

[49] Maisch B, Ristić A, Pankuweit S, Neubauer A, Moll R. Neoplastic pericardial effusion. Efficacy and safety of intrapericardial treatment with cisplatin. *European heart journal* 2002;23:1625-31.

[50] Neragi-Miandoab S, Linden PA, Ducko CT, et al. VATS pericardiotomy for patients with known malignancy and pericardial effusion: survival and prognosis of positive cytology and metastatic involvement of the pericardium: a case control study. *International Journal of Surgery* 2008;6:110-4.

[51] Moores DW, Allen KB, Faber LP, et al. Subxiphoid pericardial drainage for pericardial tamponade. *The Journal of thoracic and cardiovascular surgery* 1995;109:546-52.

In: Cardiac Tamponade
Editor: Cameron L. Pittman
ISBN: 978-1-63482-787-4

Chapter 5

Acute Dysphoria – A Mood Alteration Associated with Cardiac Tamponade

***Yuko Ikematsu*[1,*] *and Janet A. Kloos*[2]**
[1]Department of Nursing,
Nagoya University Graduate School of Medicine, Japan
[2]Medical Surgical Nursing Department, University Hospitals Case Medical Center, Cleveland, Ohio

Abstract

Cardiac tamponade is a life-threatening emergency associated with a variety of medical and surgical conditions. Since the signs and symptoms of an underlying disease are often co-manifesting, diagnosing cardiac tamponade is difficult. It is well known that cardiac tamponade patients experience mood alterations or disturbances prior to hemodynamic deterioration. Mood alterations such as being "anxious" and "restless" have been described most frequently in nursing and medical literature. A chart review study found that patients were most frequently observed as having "aggressive body movements" followed by "gets up/tries to get up" and "restless." Various kinds of facial expressions were also

* Corresponding author: E-mail: ikematsu@met.nagoya-u.ac.jp.

recorded. A short interview study of patients who had recently survived cardiac tamponade revealed that patients felt something really bad was happening, felt anxious, and couldn't stay still. Knowing characteristics of such changes in the patient's mood may help clinicians suspect cardiac tamponade. Identifying characteristic mood disturbances may facilitate further exploration of the diagnostic process including echocardiogram and may lead to timely treatment and enhanced survival.

Introduction

Nursing is defined as "the protection, promotion, and optimization of health and abilities, prevention of illness and injury, alleviation of suffering through the diagnosis and treatment of human response, and advocacy in the care of individuals, families, communities, and populations" by American Nurses Association [1]. Clinical nurses are responsible for detecting a life-threatening response to a health problem. Cardiac tamponade is one of the life-threatening complications following a variety of medical and surgical conditions. Nurses are at the front line to detect early signs and symptoms in patients experiencing cardiac tamponade. Cardiac tamponade is known to be difficult to diagnose because of its non-specific manifestation and preexisting medical conditions. [2-4] Patients with life-threatening illness including cardiac tamponade often become restless and agitated before they collapse. This mood alteration may be an important alarm for very early stage of cardiac tamponade. Knowing the mood alteration associated with cardiac tamponade may help clinicians who care for at risk patients detect an impending emergency.

Mood Alteration in Literature

Mood alteration associated with cardiac tamponade is widely mentioned in the nursing and medical literature. According to a literature review study of 100 nursing and medical textbooks and lecture journal articles [5], 42% of them included some phrases about mood alteration of cardiac tamponade patients. The most frequently used terms to describe the alteration were "restless" and "anxiety." Both were found in 16 articles. Other terms included "agitation," "confusion," "apprehension," and "a feeling of 'impending doom."

This literature review revealed that the patient experiences an unpleasant feeling which leads to restless behaviors. However, such variation of the terminology indicates that this phenomenon is not clearly defined. In order to explore the nature of the phenomenon, clear definition of the phenomenon was warranted.

Mood Alteration in Nursing Record

A chart review study followed the above mentioned literature review study. Hospital charts of 66 events of cardiac tamponade were reviewed to identify the clinicians' descriptions of the patient's complaints and behaviors [6]. The most frequently recorded behavior was unusual body movements. Behaviors were described as "aggressive" and "violent." Some patients kicked while other patients would flail their arms.

Patients experiencing cardiac tamponade also had unusual facial expressions. Facial expressions were described as harsh, severe, and apparently indicating pain. Some patients exhibited a flat or expressionless appearance.

Patients experiencing cardiac tamponade were irritable and restless. They also tried to get up or were pulling at tubes. Patients who were not intubated verbalized their feelings. Most of them described their feeling in vague words. Some patients felt somewhat strange while others felt like everything was crazy. Feeling restless was also recorded. The patients expressed such feeling as "No place to put (my) body" or "Difficult to stay still." It is noteworthy that some patients mentioned "death" which is not favorably used in health care settings in Japan. Examples of the phrases are "Will I come back alive?" and "I will die due to shortness of breath." These words may be relevant to the phrase "impending doom" frequently used in the literature.

Mood Alteration Described by Patients

Following the studies above, an interview study was conducted [7]. Patients who survived cardiac tamponade were interviewed while they were in the ICU. Three quarters of the patients affirmed that they felt "something really bad is happening" whereas more than half of the patients affirmed "feeling anxious," "could not stay still," and "difficult to settle down." Besides these precedent feelings, patients described that they experienced uncertainty, fear, ill-feeling, and an unusual sensation. This variation of the terms indicate that cardiac tamponade patients experience an uncomfortable feeling which cannot be easily described by a single word. Lack of exact terminology may hinder practical communication between the patients and heath care professionals. Therefore, definitive terms which represent the characteristics of the mood alteration of cardiac tamponade patients was warranted.

Conceptualization of the Mood Alteration

The mood alteration experienced by patients with cardiac tamponade has been conceptualized as "Dysphoria." It has been temporarily defined as "an unpleasant sensation consisting of anxiety, malaise, and a feeling of 'impending doom' manifested by restlessness, agitation, and confusion attributable to unidentified causes" based on previous studies. Although this definition is expected to be refined in successive studies, this conceptualization may help clinicians to detect early trend of cardiac tamponade in which typical signs and symptoms are still subtle.

Usefulness of Dysphoria in Clinical Settings

The sole symptom of dysphoria may not be sufficient to detect cardiac tamponade. It can be used in combination with other signs and symptoms. Dyspnea is the most prominent physical symptom in patients with cardiac tamponade [7-9]. However, most of the patients in the chart review study were well oxygenated as evidenced by high levels of saturated hemoglobin by pulse oximeter [6]. Dyspnea is a common symptom associated with a variety of diseases and conditions including congestive heart failure, pneumonia, pneumothorax, and so on. When the patient at risk for cardiac tamponade complains of dyspnea in the setting of high oxygen saturation, presence or absence of dysphoria may help clinicians to step forward to perform a definitive diagnostic procedure such as an echocardiogram. To determine whether the patient is experiencing dysphoria or not, the clinician can ask the patient if they feel like something really bad is happening, if it is difficult to settle down, of if they feel anxious. Clinicians are also advised to pay attention to the patient's harsh facial expression and restlessness.

This knowledge can be used in a wide range of specialty areas. Cardiac tamponade can be a complication of cardiovascular diseases, cancer, endocrine diseases, renal failure, and autoimmune diseases. It can also develop in patients who undergo anticoagulant therapy. Clinicians who take care of patients at risk for cardiac tamponade are encouraged to acquire assessment skills to detect early signs and symptoms of cardiac tamponade including dysphoria.

Usefulness of Dysphoria at Home

Many patients in the studies cited above developed cardiac tamponade at home. Dysphoria should be included in educational programs for patients at risk for cardiac tamponade. Home dwelling cardiac tamponade patients tend to experience dysphoria and other symptoms for considerable length of time - up to a couple of months [2, 7]. Such patients may hesitate or delay seeking an appointment with their healthcare provider because their symptoms are vague. This vagueness has been endorsed by the fact that patients reported that they felt "uncertain." [7] If such patients are educated that their vague feeling of "impending doom" and restlessness are meaningful signs to seek medical care, they may present themselves earlier and be able to receive appropriate treatment.

Family members of the potential patients should be also educated. Family members could be advised to observe the patient's facial expressions, body movements, and feelings of uncertainty or "impending doom." When the patient is indecisive in seeking medical care, family members may be able to encourage them to do so if they find the patient with a harsh facial expression, behaving restless, or having a feeling of uncertainty.

Conclusion

Although acute mood alteration of life-threatening emergencies had long been known in nursing and medicine, it was not evidence-based. Recent research studies are revealing that the mood alteration or dysphoria actually precedes hemodynamic deterioration of cardiac tamponade patients. Clinicians are recommended to utilize knowledge about the symptom of dysphoria in patients at risk for cardiac tamponade. Early detection and treatment of cardiac tamponade can be a preventative action to enhance survival.

References

[1] American Nurses Association. What is Nursing? [cited 2015 February 2]; Available from: http://www.nursingworld.org/ EspeciallyForYou/ What-is-Nursing.

[2] Larose, E; Ducharme, A; Mercier, LA; Pelletier, G; Harel, F; Tardif, JC. Prolonged distress and clinical deterioration before pericardial drainage in patients with cardiac tamponade. *The Canadian Journal of Cardiology*., 2000, 16(3), 331-6.

[3] Spodick, DH. Acute cardiac tamponade. *The New England Journal of Medicine*., 2003, 349(7), 684-90.

[4] Roosen, J; Frans, E; Wilmer, A; Knockaert, DC; Bobbaers, H. Comparison of premortem clinical diagnoses in critically ill patients and subsequent autopsy findings. *Mayo Clinic Proceedings*., 2000, 75(6), 562-7.

[5] Ikematsu, Y. Symptoms of cardiac tamponade patients in literature. *Annual Report of Sasakawa Health Science Foundation*. 1997, 5, 15-8.

[6] Ikematsu, Y. Incidence and characteristics of dysphoria in patients with cardiac tamponade. *Heart & Lung : The Journal of Critical Care*. 2007, 36(6), 440-9.

[7] Ikematsu, Y; Kloos, JA. Patients' descriptions of dysphoria associated with cardiac tamponade. *Heart & Lung : The Journal of Critical Care*., 2012, 41(3), 264-70.

[8] Gibbs, CR; Watson, RD; Singh, SP; Lip, GY. Management of pericardial effusion by drainage: a survey of 10 years' experience in a city centre general hospital serving a multiracial population. *Postgraduate Medical Journal*. 2000, 76(902), 809-13.

[9] Press, OW; Livingston, R. Management of malignant pericardial effusion and tamponade. *JAMA*., 1987, 257(8), 1088-92.

Index

C

G

H

I

J

K

L

M

Q

R

S

T

U

V

W

X